Calories, Carbohydrates & Sodium

THE NO NONSENSE
HEALTH GUIDE

Calories, Carbohydrates & Sodium

By
Harry Friend
and Louise Chapman

Cover photography by Henry Wolf/Image Bank
Cover design by Bud Lavery/
Ross Culbert Holland & Lavery, Inc.
Production services W. S. Konecky Associates, New York.

Published exclusively for Longmeadow Press, 201 High Ridge
Road, Stamford, Connecticut 06904. No part of this book may
be reproduced or used in any form or by any means,
electronic or mechanical, including photocopying, recording,
or by any information storage and retrieval system,
without permission in writing from the publisher.

ISBN: 0-681-40093-5

Printed in the United States of America

9 8 7 6 5 4 3 2 1

To Mati and Mordechai Rosenstein, whose friendship brightens every season

Introduction

The No-Nonsense Health Guide to Calories, Carbohy- *drates and Sodium* is your guidebook to thousands of basic and brand name foods. Its easy-to-read format is arranged alphabetically for quick reference. The quantities given are those you are most likely to find useful, whether at the market or in a restaurant. Like all other *No-Nonsense Guides*, this book tells you what you need to know, clearly and concisely.

Before you begin looking up various foods and their contents, take a minute to think about what you eat.

Nutrition—Know What You Eat

It helps to understand the content of the food you eat, whether or not you have a weight or other medical problem. Eating properly is essential to maintaining good health and preventing disease.

Those of us who lead busy lives often have to rely on restaurant or "convenience" foods for nutrition. This

INTRODUCTION

No-Nonsense Guide will help you understand what you're eating by listing many common food "portion" sizes and proportions for comparison and reference.

Eat a Variety of Foods

Whether or not you're on a diet, it's important to eat a variety of foods in order to maintain good health. Each day, you should eat selections from the four basic food groups: (1) fruits and vegetables, (2) breads and cereals, (3) milk, cheese and yogurt, and (4) meats, poultry, fish, eggs and legumes (dry peas and beans). Your body needs many nutrients, including vitamins, minerals, proteins and fats, to stay strong and healthy. With variety, you are less likely to develop either a deficiency or an excess of any particular nutrient.

Using This Book

This *No-Nonsense Health Guide* lists foods alphabetically by group. For example, *sirloin steak* will be found under *beef*, and *beer* under *beverages, alcoholic*. Fast food restaurants are listed by name in the overall alphabetical listing, while brand name items are listed after their generic counterparts. Major brand names are given for specific reference as well as for comparison analysis with the generic and with other brands available in your area. Use *The No-Nonsense Guide* to check and compare.

Most of the statistics given in this book for generic foods, such as asparagus or apples, rely on the analysis of the U. S. Department of Agriculture (USDA). Statistics on brand name and fast foods have been supplied by the manufacturer and are accurate as of the date of writing. Remember that these may change as manufacturers improve or modify their products.

INTRODUCTION

Portions

The weights provided in this book sometimes include inedible parts, such as skin or seeds. However, the values calculated for calories, carbohydrates and sodium are for the edible parts only.

It is important to understand the size of the portions you eat. This may sometimes require a little homework. It's often difficult to be certain of the weight of a chicken leg or a piece of roast beef.

We suggest that, in the beginning, you use a scale and measuring cup to help weigh and measure foods accurately until your eye learns to judge with precision. Don't guess. Guessing can lead to diet disaster. Also, get in the habit of reading food packages carefully. As a particular point, if you use convenience frozen dinners, always check the weights. Even when the sizes look similar, the portions (by weight) can vary tremendously.

For this reason, the portions given are those we felt were the most usable, both from a food preparation viewpoint as well as for those who eat convenience foods or in restaurants (fast or gourmet). While it is not often easy to judge the weight of a specific portion of food, it is easier, for example, to judge its size, and for that reason, the length, width and thickness of many restaurant offerings are given in addition to the weight. Of course, you could always ask the waiter/ waitress to weigh your meal, but that could prove inconvenient in many cases.

What Is a Calorie?

Calories are a measure of the energy a given food provides. A calorie is not a nutrient, but a unit of energy. Calorie measurements consider a food only as fuel to be burned, whatever the other qualities the food may have.

INTRODUCTION

One pound of fat equals 3,500 calories. So, you will gain one pound if you eat 3,500 calories more than you need to maintain your weight. And you will lose one pound if you eat 3,500 calories less. Another way of losing weight is to expend more energy, for example, by exercising. Weight control is a matter of balancing your caloric intake against the energy you expend.

What Are Carbohydrates?

Carbohydrates are one of the important components of the foods we eat. Since carbohydrates are also a source of calories, some diets recommend their reduction. Since many of the foods containing carbohydrates may carry other advantages from a health standpoint, we recommend a balanced approach in the absence of specific instructions from your doctor.

In the average diet, carbohydrates are likely to comprise between 40% and 50% of the daily caloric intake. Some doctors and nutritionists are now recommending a daily increase in foods rich in fiber and complex carbohydrates—such as fruits, vegetables, whole-grain breads and cereals. You should also note that some athletes increase their carbohydrate intake prior to competition because they believe that carbohydrates provide sustained usable energy.

What about Sodium?

There has been considerable controversy in recent years over the effects of sodium in the diet. But there is no doubt that people with hypertension (high blood pressure) or other medical conditions should consult their doctors about restricting their sodium intake.

There is less agreement as to the extent to which people without known medical problems should also limit sodium intake as a precautionary measure. The

INTRODUCTION

1986 American Heart Association revised dietary guidelines recommend that an adult should limit daily consumption of sodium to one gram (also expressed as 1,000 milligrams or 1,000 mg) of sodium for every 1,000 calories consumed, with a maximum limit of 3 grams (3,000 mg) daily. Note that one level teaspoon of table salt contains over 2,100 mg of sodium. When you look at the sodium content of many prepared and convenience foods, you will understand how easy it is for the average American, on the average American diet, to exceed these recommended limits.

Ask Your Doctor

Since your doctor is best equipped to judge your individual needs, you should ask your doctor about diet and nutrition. And before you begin any weight adjustment program, be sure to get your doctor's advice.

Abbreviations and Symbols

The following abbreviations and symbols appear in this book:

approx = approximately		pt = pint
diam = diameter		qt = quart
ex lg = extra large		sq = square
fl = fluid		tbsp = tablespoon
g = gram		tsp = teaspoon
gal = gallon		wt = weight
lb = pound		& = and
lg = large		" = inch
med = medium		< = less than
mg = milligram		− = quantity indeterminate
oz = ounce		v = varies according to brand
pkg = package		or type

INTRODUCTION

Table of Equivalents

VOLUME

$$1 \text{ quart} = 32 \text{ fluid ounces} = 4 \text{ cups}$$
$$1 \text{ quart} = 2 \text{ pints}$$
$$1 \text{ pint} = 16 \text{ fluid ounces} = 2 \text{ cups}$$
$$1 \text{ cup} = 8 \text{ fluid ounces}$$
$$1 \text{ cup} = 16 \text{ tablespoons}$$
$$1/4 \text{ cup} = 4 \text{ tablespoons}$$
$$2 \text{ tablespoons} = 1 \text{ fluid ounce}$$
$$1 \text{ tablespoon} = \frac{1}{2} \text{ fluid ounce}$$
$$3 \text{ teaspoons} = 1 \text{ tablespoon}$$
$$6 \text{ teaspoons} = 1 \text{ fluid ounce}$$

WEIGHT

$$1 \text{ pound} = 16 \text{ ounces}$$
$$1 \text{ pound} = 454 \text{ grams}$$
$$1 \text{ ounce} = 28.35 \text{ grams}$$
$$1 \text{ gram} = 1,000 \text{ milligrams}$$
$$3.52 \text{ ounces} = 100 \text{ grams}$$

Calories, Carbohydrates & Sodium

Food	Quantity or Portion	Calories	Carbo-hydrates (grams)	Sodium (milli-grams)
Acerola	10 fruits	23	5.6	7
Acerola Juice	1 cup	56	11.6	7
Ale				
See Beer				
Allspice, ground	1 tsp	5	1.4	1
Almonds				
in shell	10 nuts	60	2.0	trace
whole, shelled	1 cup	849	27.7	6
chopped	1 cup	777	25.4	5
	1 tbsp	48	1.6	.4
roasted (in oil & salted)	1 cup	984	30.6	311
	1 lb	2,844	88.5	898
	1 oz	178	5.5	56
Amaranth	1 lb	163	29.5	—
Anchovies (not heavily salted, flat	2 oz can	79	.1	—
or rolled, canned, drained)	5 anchovies	35	.1	—
Anise seed	1 tsp	7	1.05	trace
Apples				
fresh, with skin	1 fruit, 3¼″ diam, approx 2 per lb	123	30.7	2
	1 fruit, 3″ diam, approx 2½ per lb	96	24.0	2
	1 fruit, 2¾″ diam, approx 3 per lb	80	20.0	1
	1 fruit, 2½″ diam, approx 4 per lb	61	15.3	1
	1 cup quarters or finely chopped pieces	73	18.1	1
fresh, without skin	1 fruit, 3¼″ diam, approx 2 per lb	107	27.9	2
	1 fruit, 3″ diam, approx 2½ per lb	84	21.8	2
	1 fruit, 2¾″ diam, approx 3 per lb	70	18.2	1
	1 fruit, 2½″ diam, approx 4 per lb	53	13.9	1
	1 cup quarters or finely chopped pieces	68	17.6	1
dehydrated, sulfured				
uncooked	1 cup	353	92.1	7
	1 lb	1,601	417.8	32
cooked with added sugar	1 cup	194	50.0	3
	1 lb	345	88.9	5
dried, sulfured (rings)				
uncooked	8 oz container	624	163.0	11
	1 cup	234	61.0	4
	1 lb	1,247	325.7	23
cooked				
without added sugar	1 cup	199	51.8	3
	1 lb	354	92.1	5

Food	Quantity or Portion	Calories	Carbo-hydrates (grams)	Sodium (milli-grams)
with added sugar	1 cup	314	81.8	3
	1 lb	508	132.5	5
frozen, sliced, sweetened with nutritive sweetener, not thawed	1 lb	422	110.2	299
Apple Brown Betty	1 cup	325	63.9	329
Apple Butter	12 oz jar	632	159.1	7
	1 cup	525	132.0	6
	1 tbsp	33	8.2	trace
Apple Juice	5½ fl oz can	80	20.3	2
	1 cup	177	29.5	2
	6 oz glass	87	22.1	2
	1 fl oz	15	3.7	trace
Applesauce, canned				
unsweetened	1 lb can	186	49.0	9
	1 cup	100	26.4	5
sweetened with nutritive sweetener	1 lb can	426	111.4	9
	1 cup	232	60.7	5
Apricots				
raw, whole	1 lb (approx 12)	217	54.6	4
	3 apricots	55	13.7	1
raw, halves	1 lb	231	58.1	5
	1 cup	79	19.8	2
canned, fruit & liquid				
water packed without artificial sweetener, halved style	1 lb can (12–20 halves) with approx 9½ tbsp liquid	172	43.5	5
	1 cup	93	23.6	2
	3 halves, 1¾ tbsp liquid	32	8.1	1
heavy syrup packed (whole apricots with pits or halves, pitted)	17 oz can whole style (8–14 apricots)	390	99.7	5
	17 oz can, halved style (12–20 halves)	415	106.0	5
	1 cup, either style	222	56.9	3
	3 halves, 1¾ tbsp liquid	73	18.7	1
dehydrated, sulfured, nugget type & pieces				
uncooked	1 cup	332	84.6	33
	1 lb	1,506	383.7	150
cooked, fruit & liquid, sugar added	1 cup	337	91.5	24
	1 lb	540	138.3	36
dried, sulfured (lg halves, 1½″ diam; med halves, 1⅛″ diam)				
uncooked	11 oz container	811	207.5	81
	1 cup	338	86.5	34
	10 halves, lg	125	31.9	12
	10 halves, med	91	23.3	9

Food	Quantity or Portion	Calories	Carbohydrates (grams)	Sodium (milligrams)
cooked, fruit & liquid				
without added sugar	1 cup	213	54.0	20
	1 lb	386	98.0	36
with added sugar	1 cup	329	84.8	19
	1 lb	553	142.4	32
frozen, sweetened	1 lb	445	113.9	18
Apricot nectar	5½ oz can	99	25.3	trace
	6 oz glass	107	27.4	trace
	1 cup	143	36.6	trace
Arby's				
Roast Beef				
Junior	3 oz	218	22	345
Regular	5.2 oz	353	32	590
Beef 'N Cheddar	6.7 oz	490	51	1,520
Bac 'N Cheddar Deluxe	8 oz	561	36	1,385
King	6.7 oz	467	44	765
Super	8.3 oz	501	50	800
Chicken Breast Sandwich	7.4 oz	592	56	1,340
Hot Ham 'N Cheese Sandwich	5.7 oz	353	33	1,655
Turkey Deluxe	7 oz	375	32	850
Potatoes				
Plain	11 oz	290	66	12
Deluxe	11 oz	648	59	475
Broccoli & Cheddar	12 oz	541	72	475
Mushroom & Cheese	10.5 oz	506	61	635
French Fries	2.5 oz	211	33	30
Potato Cakes	3 oz	201	22	425
Taco	15 oz	619	73	1,065
Shakes				
Chocolate	10.6 oz	384	62	300
Jamocha	10.8	424	76	280
Vanilla	8.8 oz	295	44	245
Artichokes, globe or French,	1 lg artichoke	67(a)	15.0	46
cooked (boiled), drained (a)	1 small artichoke	44(a)	9.9	30
Asparagus				
raw, spears (green)	1 cup, 1½–2" pieces	35	6.8	3
	1 lb	118	22.7	9
cooked spears (green), boiled,	4 lg spears	20	3.6	1
drained, added salt	4 med spears	12	2.2	1
	4 small spears	8	1.4	trace
	1 cup, 1½–2" cut pieces	29	5.2	1
canned, (green) regular pack				
asparagus & liquid	10½ oz can	74	11.9	970
	1 cup, whole spears with liquid	44	7.1	576
	1 cup, cut spears with liquid	43	6.9	564

(a) Values for stored artichokes. Caloric values may be as little as 50% or even 25% of those stated if freshly harvested artichokes are used.

Food	Quantity or Portion	Calories	Carbo-hydrates (grams)	Sodium (milli-grams)
drained asparagus	4 spears, each ½" diam at base	17	2.7	189
	4 spears, ⅜" diam at base	13	2.0	142
	1 cup whole spears	51	8.2	571
	1 cup cut spears	49	8.0	555
canned, green, special dietary pack (low sodium)				
asparagus & liquid, cut spears	14½ oz can	66	11.1	12
	1 cup	38	6.5	7
	1 lb	73	12.2	14
drained asparagus (cut spears)	1 cup	47	7.3	7
	1 lb	91	14.1	14
canned, white (bleached), regular pack				
asparagus & liquid	10½ oz can	54	9.8	703
	1 cup, whole spears	44	8.1	576
	1 cup, cut spears	43	7.9	564
drained asparagus	1 cup, whole spears	53	8.7	571
	1 cup, cut spears	52	8.5	555
	4 spears, each ½" diam at base	18	2.9	189
	4 spears, each ⅜" diam at base	13	2.2	142
canned, white, special dietary pack (low sodium)				
asparagus & liquid (cut spears)	14½ oz can	66	12.3	16
	1 cup	38	7.2	10
drained asparagus (cut spears)	1 cup	45	8.2	9
	1 lb	86	15.9	18
frozen (green), boiled & drained	4 lg (¾" diam) spears	18	3.0	1
	4 med (½" diam) spears	14	2.3	1
	4 small (⅜" diam) spears	9	1.5	trace
	1 cup spears	44	7.2	2
Avocados, raw	whole fruit, 10⅔ oz	378	14.3	9
	½ fruit, served with skin	188	7.1	5
	1 cup cubes (½")	251	9.5	6
	1 cup, puree (mashed or sieved)	384	14.5	9

B

Baby Food, brand names
 Beech-Nut

Food	Quantity or Portion	Calories	Carbo-hydrates	Sodium
Applesauce	4½ oz	60	14	5
Bananas	4½ oz	100	24	5

Food	Quantity or Portion	Calories	Carbo-hydrates (grams)	Sodium (milli-grams)
Beef	3½ oz	120	1	75
Carrots	4½ oz	40	8	130
Chicken	3½ oz	110	1	70
Green Beans	4½ oz	40	8	10
Lamb	3½ oz	130	1	80
Peaches	4½ oz	60	14	5
Pears	4½ oz	70	16	5
Peas	4½ oz	70	12	5
Squash	4½ oz	30	7	10
Sweet Potatoes	4½ oz	70	16	60
Turkey	3½ oz	120	1	60
Veal	3½ oz	120	1	70
Beech-Nut Juice				
Orange	4.2 fl oz	60	14	5
Beech-Nut Junior Foods				
Apricots	7½ oz	120	29	10
Bananas	7½ oz	160	38	10
Chicken Noodle Dinner	7½ oz	140	23	50
Peaches	7½ oz	150	37	10
Pears	7½ oz	140	35	10
Turkey Rice Dinner	7½ oz	120	20	60
Vanilla Custard Pudding	7½ oz	200	36	100
Vegetable Bacon Dinner	7½ oz	180	22	200
Vegetable Beef Dinner	7½ oz	130	20	90
Enfamil and Enfamil with Iron	5 fl oz, prepared as directed	100	10.3	27
Gerber, strained				
Applesauce	4½ oz	60	14	0
Apricot with Tapioca	4½ oz	100	21	15
Bananas	4½ oz	100	21	15
Carrots	4½ oz	40	7	140
Cherry Vanilla Pudding	4½ oz	90	21	20
Chicken	4½ oz	140	1	55
Creamed Spinach	4½ oz	60	10	135
Mixed Cereal with Applesauce & Bananas	4½ oz	100	22	<20
Mixed Vegetables	4½ oz	50	10	25
Oatmeal	4½ oz	100	22	<20
Peaches	4½ oz	90	20	15
Pears	4½ oz	80	16	0
Peas	4½ oz	60	10	10
Rice Cereal	4½ oz	100	23	25
Sweet Potatoes	4½ oz	80	18	60
Vegetable Beef Dinner	4½ oz	80	11	35
Vegetable Chicken Dinner	4½ oz	80	12	30
Gerber Strained Juices				
Apple	1 bottle	60	15	0
Mixed Fruit	1 bottle	60	14	10
Orange	1 bottle	70	14	<20
Gerber Cereal				
High Protein	½ oz (4 tbsp)	50	6	<20
Mixed Cereal	½ oz (4 tbsp)	60	10	0
Rice Cereal	½ oz (4 tbsp)	60	11	0

Food	Quantity or Portion	Calories	Carbo-hydrates (grams)	Sodium (milli-grams)
Gerber Junior Foods				
Applesauce	7½ oz	100	23	<20
Bananas	7½ oz	150	34	25
Chicken Noodle	7½ oz	120	18	115
Peaches	7½ oz	140	32	25
Pear Pineapple	7½ oz	120	26	<20
Vegetable Beef Dinner	7½ oz	140	21	90
Vegetable Chicken Dinner	7½ oz	120	18	95
Vegetable Turkey Dinner	7½ oz	120	19	85
Heinz, strained				
Bananas with Tapioca	4½ oz	100	24	20
Heinz Instant Baby Food				
Creamed Corn	½ oz (6 tbsp)	60	10	0
Mixed Vegetables	½ oz (5 tbsp)	60	9	15
Squash	½ oz (5 tbsp)	50	10	(a)
Heinz Instant Cereal—Barley	½ oz	60	10	5
Nabisco National Arrowroot Biscuit	1 biscuit	20	3	15
Similac, prepared as directed				
Low Iron	5 oz	100	10.7	32
With Iron	5 fl oz	100	10.7	32
With Whey & Iron	5 fl oz	100	72.3	230
Bacon, cooked (broiled or fried), drained	2 thick slices, (1.3 oz each, before cooking)	143	.8	245
	2 med sliced (.8 oz each, before cooking)	86	.5	153
	2 thin slices (.6 oz each, before cooking)	61	.3	102
canned (a)	1 lb can (17–18 slices)	3,107	4.5	3,084
Bacon, Canadian style, broiled or fried, drained	yield from 6 oz (approx 6 slices)	349	.4	3,125
	¾ lb, yield from 1 lb raw	921	1.0	8,578
	1 slice	58	.1	537
Baking Powder				
sodium aluminum sulfate				
with monocalcium phosphate	1 tbsp	14	3.4	1,205
monohydrate	1 tsp	4	.9	329
with monocalcium phosphate	1 tbsp	9	2.1	1,278
monohydrate & calcium carbonate	1 tsp	2	.6	349
with monocalcium phosphate	1 tbsp	11	2.6	1,050
monohydrate & calcium sulfate	1 tsp	3	.7	290
straight phosphate	1 tbsp	15	3.7	1,028
	1 tsp	5	1.1	312
tartrate (cream of tartar with tartaric acid)	1 tbsp	7	1.8	694
	1 tsp	2	.5	204
special low-sodium preparations	1 tbsp	23	5.6	1
	1 tsp	7	1.8	trace

(a) Sodium content less than 10mg per 100g

BEANS

Food	Quantity or Portion	Calories	Carbo-hydrates (grams)	Sodium (milli-grams)
Bamboo shoots, raw	1 lb, about 3 cups	122	23.6	—
Bananas, common, raw	1 lg	116	30.2	1
	1 med	101	26.4	1
	1 small	81	21.1	1
	1 lb	386	100.7	5
	1 cup sliced	128	33.3	2
	1 cup mashed	191	50.0	2
Bananas, red	1 whole	118	30.7	1
	1 lb	408	106.1	5
Banana flakes	1 cup	340	88.6	4
(dehydrated)	1 tbsp	21	5.5	trace
	1 oz	96	25.1	1
Bananas, baking type				
See Plantain				
Barbados Cherry				
See Acerola				
Barbecue sauce	1 cup	288	20.0	2,038
Barley, pearled				
Light	1 cup	608	157.6	6
Pot or Scotch	1 cup	696	154.4	—
Basil, ground	1 tsp	4	0.85	trace
Bass, black sea, baked, stuffed	1 lb	1,175	51.7	—
	1 oz	73	3.2	—
Bass, striped, oven fried	16⅞ oz (yield from 1 lb raw fillets)	941	32.2	—
	1 fillet, 8¾" long, 4½" wide, ⅝" thick	392	13.4	—
	1 lb	889	30.4	—
	1 oz	56	1.9	—
Bay Leaf, crumbled	1 tsp	8	0.45	trace
Beans, broad				
See Broadbeans				
Beans, common, mature seeds, dry				
White				
all varieties	1 lb, raw	1,542	278.1	86
Great Northern	1 cup raw	612	110.3	34
	1 cup cooked & drained	212	38.2	13
pea (navy)	1 cup raw	697	125.7	39
	1 cup cooked & drained	224	40.3	13
canned, with pork & tomato sauce	1 lb, 4 oz can	692	107.7	2,625
	1 cup	311	48.5	1,181
canned, with pork & sweet sauce	1 lb, 4 oz can	851	119.6	2,155
	1 cup	383	53.8	969
canned, without pork	1 lb, 4 oz can	680	130.4	1,916
	1 cup	306	58.7	862
Red Kidney	1 lb raw	1,556	280.8	45
	1 cup raw	635	114.5	19
	1 cup, cooked & drained	218	39.6	6

Food	Quantity or Portion	Calories	Carbo-hydrates (grams)	Sodium (milli-grams)
canned, beans & liquid	1 lb, 4 oz can	510	93.0	17
	1 cup	230	41.8	8
Pinto, Calico, Red Mexican	1 lb, raw	1,583	288.9	45
	1 cup Pinto, raw	663	121.0	19
Black, Brown, Bayo	1 lb, raw	1,538	277.6	113
	1 cup, raw	676	122.4	50
Beans, Lima (immature seeds)	1 lb, raw	558	100.2	9
	1 cup, raw	191	34.3	3
	1 lb, boiled & drained	503	89.8	5
	1 cup, boiled & drained	189	33.7	2
canned, regular pack, beans & liquid	1 lb can	322	60.8	1,070
	1 cup	176	33.2	585
canned, regular pack, drained beans	11 oz can	300	57.1	736
	1 cup	163	31.1	401
canned, special dietary pack (low sodium), beans & liquid	1 lb can	318	58.5	18
	1 cup	174	32.0	10
canned, special dietary pack (low sodium), drained beans	1 lb can	296	55.2	12
	1 cup	162	30.1	7
frozen				
Fordhooks, (thick-seeded), boiled & drained	10 oz frozen	283	54.3	285
	1 lb frozen	452	86.7	456
	1 cup	168	32.5	172
Baby limas (thin-seeded), boiled & drained	10 oz frozen	339	64.0	367
	1 lb frozen	541	102.2	587
	1 cup	212	40.1	232
Beans, Limas, mature seeds, dry				
Fordhooks	1 cup, raw	621	115.2	7
Baby Limas	1 cup, raw	656	121.6	8
	1 lb, cooked	626	116.1	9
	1 cup	262	48.6	4
Bean Flour, Lima	1 lb	1,556	285.8	—
	1 cup, sifted	432	79.4	—
Beans, Mung				
mature seeds, dry, raw	1 lb	1,542	273.5	27
	1 cup	714	126.6	13
sprouted seeds				
uncooked	1 lb	159	29.9	23
	1 cup	37	6.9	5
boiled & drained	1 lb	127	23.6	18
	1 cup	35	6.5	5
Beans, Snap Beans, Green (String Beans)				
raw, cut	1 lb	145	32.2	32
	1 cup	35	7.8	8
boiled & drained (cuts & French style)	1 lb	113	24.5	18
	1 cup	31	6.8	5
canned, regular pack				
beans & liquid	15½ oz can	79	18.4	1,036
	1 cup	43	10.0	564

Food	Quantity or Portion	Calories	Carbo-hydrates (grams)	Sodium (milli-grams)
drained beans	1 cup, cuts	32	7.0	319
	1 cup, French style	31	6.8	307
canned, special dietary pack, low sodium				
beans & liquid	15½ oz can	70	15.8	9
	1 cup	38	8.6	5
drained beans	1 cup	30	6.5	3
frozen, cut, boiled & drained	1 lb	113	25.9	5
	1 cup	34	7.7	1
frozen, French style, boiled &	1 lb	118	27.2	9
drained	1 cup	34	7.8	3
Beans, Snap Beans, Yellow or Wax				
raw	1 lb	122	27.2	32
	1 cup	30	6.6	8
cooked, boiled & drained	1 lb	100	20.9	14
	1 cup	28	5.8	4
canned, regular pack				
beans & liquid	15½ oz can	83	18.4	1,036
	1 cup	45	10.0	564
drained beans	1 cup, cuts	32	7.0	319
	1 cup, French style	31	6.8	307
canned, special dietary pack, low sodium				
beans & liquid	15½ oz can	66	14.9	9
	1 cup	36	8.1	5
drained beans	1 cup	28	6.3	3
frozen, cut, boiled & drained	1 lb	122	28.1	5
	1 cup	36	8.4	1
Beans, Baked, canned, brand names				
B&M Baked Beans	8 oz	330	49	770
Van Camp Baked Beans	8 oz	260	52	1,020
Bean Sprouts				
See Mung Beans or Soybeans				
Beans & Frankfurters				
sliced & canned	15½ oz can	632	55.3	2,366
	1 cup	367	32.1	1,374
Beaver, roasted	3 oz	211	0	—
	1 lb	1,125	0	—
Beechnuts	1 lb, in shell	1,527	56.2	—
	1 lb,, shelled	2,576	92.1	—
Beef (a)				
Boneless Chuck for stew, cooked (braised or stewed)	10.7 oz cooked (yield from 1 lb raw)	994	0	138
lean with fat	1 lb, cooked	1,483	0	206
	¼ lb, cooked	371	0	52

(a) Beef values are determined as trimmed to lean retail basis, USDA choice. (Use of lower grades will result in some calorie reduction due to lower fat content.) Cooked values refer to meat cooked without additional salt. All measures not tightly packed unless otherwise indicated.

Food	Quantity or Portion	Calories	Carbo-hydrates (grams)	Sodium (milli-grams)
	1 cup, cooked, chopped pieces	458	0	64
lean only, trimmed of separable fat	10.7 oz, cooked (yield from 1 lb raw)	651	0	160
	1 lb, cooked	971	0	238
	1 cup, cooked, chopped pieces	300	0	74
Rib Roast, choice grade, roasted lean with fat	10¾ oz, yield from 1 lb raw with bone	1,342	0	149
	11.7 oz, yield from 1 lb raw without bone	1,456	0	161
	1 lb, cooked	1,996	0	221
	¼ lb, cooked	499	0	55
lean, trimmed of separable fat	6.9 oz, yield from 1 lb raw with bone	470	0	135
	7½ oz, yield from 1 lb raw without bone	511	0	147
	1 lb, cooked	1,093	0	313
	¼ lb, cooked	273	0	78
Rump Roast, choice grade, roasted lean with fat	9.9 oz, yield from 1 lb raw with bone	975	0	162
	11.7 oz, yield from 1 lb raw without bone	1,149	0	191
	1 lb, cooked	1,574	0	262
	¼ lb, cooked	394	0	66
	1 cup, not packed, chopped or diced	486	0	81
lean, trimmed of separable fat	7.4 oz, yield from 1 lb raw with bone	439	0	150
	8.8 oz, yield from 1 lb raw without bone	516	0	177
	1 lb, cooked	943	0	323
	¼ lb, cooked	236	0	81
	1 cup, not packed, chopped or diced	291	0	100
Steak, Club, choice grade, broiled lean with fat	9.8 oz, yield from 1 lb raw with bone	1,262	0	140
	11.7 oz, yield from 1 lb raw without bone	1,503	0	167
	1 lb, cooked	2,059	0	229
	¼ lb, cooked	515	0	57
lean, trimmed of separable fat	5.7 oz, yield from 1 lb raw with bone	393	0	117
	6.8 oz, yield from 1 lb raw without bone	468	0	139

Food	Quantity or Portion	Calories	Carbo-hydrates (grams)	Sodium (milli-grams)
	1 lb, cooked	1,107	0	329
	¼ lb, cooked	277	0	82
Steak, Porterhouse, choice grade, broiled				
lean with fat	10.6 oz, yield from 1 lb raw with bone	1,400	0	145
	1 lb, cooked	2,109	0	219
	¼ lb, cooked	527	0	55
lean, trimmed of separable fat	6.1 oz, yield from 1 lb raw with bone	385	0	127
	1 lb, cooked	1,016	0	336
	¼ lb, cooked	254	0	84
Steak, Round, cooked (braised, broiled, or sauteed)				
lean with fat	10.7 oz, yield from 1 lb raw with bone	793	0	213
	11.1 oz, yield from 1 lb raw without bone	820	0	220
	1 lb, cooked	1,184	0	318
	¼ lb, cooked	296	0	80
lean, trimmed of separable fat	9.2 oz, yield from 1 lb raw with bone	491	0	199
	9½ oz, yield from 1 lb raw without bone	507	0	206
	1 lb, cooked	857	0	348
	¼ lb, cooked	214	0	87
Steak, Sirloin (double bone), choice grade, broiled				
lean with fat	9.6 oz, yield from 1 lb raw with bone	1,110	0	148
	11.7 oz, yield from 1 lb raw without bone	1,350	0	180
	1 lb, cooked	1,851	0	247
	¼ lb, cooked	463	0	62
lean, trimmed of separable fat	6.3 oz, yield from 1 lb raw with bone	387	0	134
	7.7 oz, yield from 1 lb raw without bone	471	0	163
	1 lb, cooked	980	0	340
	¼ lb, cooked	245	0	85
Steak, T-Bone, choice grade, broiled				
lean with fat	10.4 oz, yield from 1 lb raw with bone	1,395	0	141
	1 lb, cooked	2,146	0	217
	¼ lb, cooked	537	0	54
lean, trimmed of separable fat	5.8 oz, yield from 1 lb raw with bone	368	0	123
	1 lb, cooked	1,012	0	338
	¼ lb, cooked	253	0	85

Food	Quantity or Portion	Calories	Carbo-hydrates (grams)	Sodium (milli-grams)
Ground Beef, cooked (well done, oven broiled, pan broiled or sauteed)				
lean with 10% fat	12 oz, yield from 1 lb raw	745	0	228
	3 oz patty, yield from ¼ lb raw	186	0	57
lean with 21% fat	11½ oz, yield from 1 lb raw	932	0	193
	2.9 oz patty, yield from ¼ lb raw	235	0	49
Beef & Vegetable Stew				
home cooked using lean beef	1 lb	404	28.1	168
chuck	1 cup	218	15.2	91
canned	15 oz can	336	30.2	1,747
	1 cup	194	17.4	1,007
Beef, Corned, Boneless	10.7 oz, yield from 1 lb, uncooked	1,131	0	2,867
	1 lb, cooked	1,687	0	4,277
	¼ lb	422	0	1,069
canned	1 lb	980	0	—
Corned Beef Hash, canned with	1 cup	398	23.5	1,188
potato	1 lb	821	48.5	2,449
Beef, Dried, Chipped				
uncooked	1 lb	921	0	19,505
	1 oz	58	0	1,219
cooked, creamed	1 lb	699	32.2	8,248
	1 cup	377	17.4	1,754
Beef Frozen Dinners				
See Frozen Dinners				
Beef, Potted				
See Sausage, cold cuts, and luncheon meats				
Beef Potpie, home prepared	1 lb	1,116	85.3	1,288
	1 piece (⅓ pie)	517	39.5	596
Beef, sliced & frozen for steak sandwiches				
See Steak, sliced, frozen, brand name				
Beer				
See Beverages				
Beets, common red				
raw, peeled	1 cup, diced	58	13.4	81
	1 lb, diced or whole	195	44.9	272
cooked (boiled)	1 cup diced or sliced	54	12.2	73
	1 lb (approx 2⅔ cups, diced or sliced)	145	32.7	195
canned, regular pack				
beets & liquid	1 lb can	154	35.8	1,070
	1 cup	84	19.4	581

Food	Quantity or Portion	Calories	Carbo-hydrates (grams)	Sodium (milli-grams)
drained beets	1 cup, diced or sliced	63	15.0	401
	1 cup whole (small)	59	14.1	378
canned, special dietary pack, low sodium				
beets & liquid	1 lb can	145	35.4	209
	1 cup	79	19.2	113
drained beets	1 cup, diced or sliced	63	14.8	78
	1 cup, whole small	59	13.9	74
Beet Greens, common edible leaves & stems				
raw	1 lb	109	20.9	590
cooked (boiled & drained)	1 lb	82	15.0	345
	1 cup	26	4.8	110
Beverages, Alcoholic				
Beer (4.5% alcohol by volume;	12 fl oz can	151	13.7	25
3.6% by wt)	1 glass—8 fl oz	101	9.1	17
Beer, Light, Brand Names				
Bud Light	12 fl oz	108	8.8	—
Lite (Miller)	12 fl oz	96	2.8	—
Michelob Light	12 fl oz	134	12.4	—
Gin, Rum, Vodka, Whiskey				
80 proof (33.4% alcohol by wt)	1 jigger (1½ fl oz)	97	trace	trace
	1 fl oz	65	trace	trace
86 proof (36.0% alcohol by wt)	1 jigger (1½ fl oz)	105	trace	trace
	1 fl oz	70	trace	trace
90 proof (37.9% alcohol by wt)	1 jigger (1½ fl oz)	110	trace	trace
	1 fl oz	74	trace	trace
94 proof (39.7% alcohol by wt)	1 jigger (1½ fl oz)	116	trace	trace
	1 fl oz	77	trace	trace
100 proof (42.5% alcohol by wt)	1 jigger (1½ fl oz)	124	trace	trace
	1 fl oz	83	trace	trace
Wines				
Dessert (18.8% alcohol by volume; 15.3% by wt)	1 wine glass (3½ fl oz)	141	7.9	4
	1 sherry glass (2 fl oz)	81	4.5	2
	1 fl oz	41	2.3	1
Table (12.2% alcohol by volume, 9.9% by wt)	1 wine glass (3½ fl oz)	87	4.3	5
	1 fl oz	25	1.2	1
Beverages, Carbonated, nonalcoholic				
Club soda	12 oz bottle or can	0	0	—
Cola type	12 oz bottle or can	144	36.9	—
	1 fl oz	12	3.1	—
Cream Sodas	12 oz bottle or can	160	40.8	—
	1 fl oz	13	3.4	—
Fruit Flavored Sodas (citrus, cherry, grape, strawberry, Tom Collins Mixer, other) (10–13% sugar)	12 oz bottle or can	171	44.6	—
	1 fl oz	14	3.7	—
Ginger Ale, pale dry and golden	12 oz bottle or can	113	29.3	—
	1 fl oz	9	2.4	—

Food	Quantity or Portion	Calories	Carbo-hydrates (grams)	Sodium (milli-grams)
Quinine sodas	12 oz bottle or can	113	29.3	—
	1 fl oz	9	2.4	—
Root Beer	12 oz bottle or can	152	38.9	—
	1 fl oz	13	3.2	—
Special Dietary Drinks with artificial sweetener (less than 1 calorie per oz)	12 oz bottle or can	1	—	—
Beverages, nonalcoholic—by brand name				
Gatorade				
Lemon-Lime	8 fl oz	50	14	110
Orange	8 fl oz	50	14	110
Fruit Punch	8 fl oz	50	14	110
Country Time Sugar Free				
all flavors	8 fl oz	4	0	0
Crystal Light Sugar Free				
all flavors	8 fl oz	4	0	0
Hawaiian Punch				
Fruit Juicy Red	6 fl oz	90	22	20
Island Fruit Cocktail	6 fl oz	90	22	30
Red Grape Punch	6 fl oz	90	23	30
Tropical Fruit	6 fl oz	90	22	30
Very Berry	6 fl oz	90	22	30
Wild Fruit	6 fl oz	90	23	35
Hi C				
Candy Apple Cooler	6 fl oz	90	23	20
Cherry	6 fl oz	100	25	25
Citrus Cooler	6 fl oz	100	24	20
Double Fruit Cooler	6 fl oz	90	23	20
Fruit Punch	6 fl oz	100	24	20
Grape Drink	6 fl oz	100	24	25
Hula Cooler	6 fl oz	100	24	20
Orange Drink	6 fl oz	100	24	20
Peach	6 fl oz	100	25	20
Strawberry	6 fl oz	100	24	20
Wild Berry	6 fl oz	90	23	20
Kool-Aid				
all flavors, unsweetened	8 fl oz	2	0	0
all flavors, sweetened	8 fl oz	100	25	0
Sugar-Free	8 fl oz	4	0	—
Sunkist Light Sugar Free				
Lemonade flavor	8 fl oz	8	2	35
Orange flavor	8 fl oz	8	2	70
V-8 Juice	6 fl oz	35	8	640
Biscuits, baking powder, home baked, made with enriched or un-enriched flour	1 biscuit 2″ diam	103	12.8	175
	1 lb	1,674	207.7	2,840
From Biscuit mix with enriched flour, made with milk	1 biscuit 2″ diam	91	14.6	272
	1 lb	1,474	237.2	4,414
Blackberries (including Dewberries, Boysenberries & Youngberries)	1 cup, raw	84	18.6	1

Food	Quantity or Portion	Calories	Carbo-hydrates (grams)	Sodium (milli-grams)
Blackberries, canned, berries & liquid				
Water pack without artificial	1 cup	98	22.0	2
sweetener	1 lb	181	40.8	5
Syrup pack, heavy	1 lb can	413	100.7	5
Blackberries, frozen				
See Boysenberries				
Blackberry juice, canned, unsweetened	1 cup	91	19.1	2
Blackeye Peas				
See Cowpeas				
Blancmange				
See Puddings				
Blueberries				
raw	1 pt	254	62.7	4
	1 cup	90	22.2	1
	1 lb	281	69.4	5
frozen, not thawed	10 oz, unsweetened	156	38.6	3
	1 cup, unsweetened	91	22.4	2
	10 oz, sweetened with nutritive sweetener	298	75.3	3
	1 cup, sweetened with nutritive sweetener	242	61.0	2
Bluefish, cooked (Baked or broiled with butter or margarine)	12⅞ oz (yield from 1 lb fillets)	580	0	380
	1 oz	45	0	29
fried	13⅜ oz (yield from 1 lb fillets)	789	18.1	562
	1 oz	58	1.3	41
Bockwurst				
See Sausage, cold cuts & luncheon meats				
Bologna				
See Sausage, cold cuts and luncheon meats				
Boston Brown Bread, canned	1 lb can	957	206.8	1,139
Bouillon cubes or powder (instant)	1 cube (½″)	5	.2	960
	1 packet powder (2½ tsp)	6	.3	1,200
	1 tsp	2	.1	480
Boysenberries				
canned, water pack, berries &	1 cup	88	22.2	2
liquid, without artificial sweetener	1 lb	163	41.3	5
frozen, not thawed, unsweetened	10 oz container	136	32.4	3
	1 cup	60	14.4	1
frozen, not thawed, with nutritive	10 oz container	273	69.3	3
sweetener	1 cup	137	34.9	1
Bran				
with added sugar, salt, malt extract, vitamins	1 cup	144	44.6	493

Food	Quantity or Portion	Calories	Carbo-hydrates (grams)	Sodium (milli-grams)
with added sugar, salt, defatted wheat germ, vitamins	1 cup	179	59.1	368
Bran Flakes (40% bran) with added sugar, salt, iron, vitamins	1 cup	106	28.2	207
Bran Flakes with raisins, added sugar, salt, iron, vitamins	1 cup	144	39.7	212
Braunschweiger				
See Sausage, cold cuts, & luncheon meats				
Brazil nuts				
in shell	1 cup (approx 13½ lg nuts)	383	6.4	1
	1 oz (3 ex lg or 3½ lg nuts)	89	1.5	trace
shelled	1 cup (32 lg nuts)	916	15.3	1
	1 oz (6 ex lg or lg or 8 med nuts)	185	3.1	trace
Breads				
See also Biscuits, Boston Brown Bread, Cornbread, Muffins, Rolls, Salt Sticks				
Cracked Wheat	1 lb loaf	1,193	236.3	2,400
	1 slice (1/18 loaf)	66	13.0	132
French or Vienna Bread & rolls, enriched or unenriched				
bread	1 lb loaf	1,315	251.3	2,631
slice, French	5 × 2½ × 1″	102	19.4	203
	2½ × 2 × ½″	44	8.3	87
slice, Vienna	4¾ × 4 × ½″	73	13.9	145
roll, hoagie or submarine, 11½ × 3 × 2½″	1 roll	392	74.8	783
Italian Bread, enriched or unenriched				
bread	1 lb loaf	1,252	255.8	2,645
slice	4½ × 3¼ × ¾″	83	16.9	176
slice	3¼ × 2½ × ½″	28	5.6	59
Melba Toast				
See Melba Toast				
Raisin Bread				
bread	1 lb loaf	1,188	243.1	1,656
slice	1/18 loaf	66	13.4	91
Rye Bread				
American (⅔ wheat flour, ⅓ rye flour)				
bread	1 lb loaf	1,102	236.3	2,527
slice	1/18 loaf	61	13.0	139
snack size	8 oz loaf	552	118.3	1,264
	¼″ slice	17	3.6	39
Pumpernickel				
bread	1 lb loaf	1,116	240.9	2,581
slice	1/14 loaf	79	17.0	182

Food	Quantity or Portion	Calories	Carbo-hydrates (grams)	Sodium (milli-grams)
snack size	8 oz loaf	558	120.5	1,292
	¼″ slice	17	3.7	40
Salt-rising Bread, unenriched				
bread	1 lb loaf	1,211	236.8	1,202
slice	⅛ loaf	64	12.5	64
White bread, enriched or unen-riched (a)				
bread	1 lb loaf	1,225	229.1	2,300
slice	⅛ loaf	68	12.6	127
thin slice	½₂ loaf	54	10.1	101
	1 cup cubes	81	15.2	152
	1 cup crumbs	122	22.7	228
Whole Wheat Bread (a)				
bread	1 lb loaf	1,102	216.4	2,390
slice	⅛ loaf	61	11.9	132
slice	½₀ loaf	56	11.0	121
Breads, Frozen				
See Croissants				
Breadcrumbs, dry, grated	1 cup	392	73.4	736
Breadcrumbs and cubes				
See Bread, White				
Bread Pudding with Raisins (a)	1 cup	496	75.3	533
Bread Sticks				
See Salt Sticks, regular type				
Bread stuffings prepared from mix				
Mix, dry form	8 oz pkg	842	164.3	3,021
	1 cup coarse crumbs	260	50.7	932
	1 cup cubes	111	21.7	399
Stuffing				
dry, crumbly, prepared with	1 cup	501	49.8	1,254
water, table fat	1 lb	1,624	161.5	4,064
moist, prepared with water,	1 cup	416	39.4	1,008
egg, table fat	1 lb	943	89.4	2,286
Breakfast cereals				
See Corn, Oats, Rice, Wheat, also Bran, Farina				
Broadbeans, raw	1 lb immature seeds	476	80.7	18
	1 lb mature seeds dry	1,533	264.0	—
Broccoli, stalks (head or bud clus-ters, stem & leaves)				
raw	1 lb (2 lg, 3 med or 4 small stalks)	145	26.8	68
cooked (boiled), drained				
stalks, whole	1 lg stalk	73	12.6	28
	1 med stalk	47	8.1	18
	1 small stalk	36	6.3	14
	1 cup, cut	40	7.0	16
frozen				
chopped, cooked (boiled), drained	yield from 10 oz frozen (1⅜ cups)	65	11.5	38

(a) Content may vary slightly according to baker.

Food	Quantity or Portion	Calories	Carbo-hydrates (grams)	Sodium (milli-grams)
	yield from 1 lb frozen (2¹⁄₁₆ cups)	104	18.4	60
	1 cup	48	8.5	28
spears or stalks, cooked (boiled), drained	yield from 10 oz frozen (7–9 spears)	65	11.8	30
	yield from 1 lb frozen (11–14 spears)	104	18.8	48
	1 spear or stalk	8	1.4	4
Brown Betty				
See Apple Brown Betty				
Brownies				
See Cookies				
Brussel Sprouts				
raw	1 lb (about 24 sprouts)	204	37.6	64
cooked, (boiled), drained	1 cup (7–8 sprouts)	56	9.9	16
	4 sprouts	30	5.4	8
	1 lb (24 sprouts)	163	29.0	45
frozen, cooked (boiled), drained	yield from 10 oz frozen (1¾–1⅞ cups)	94	18.5	40
	yield from 1 lb frozen (2⅞–3 cups)	150	29.6	64
	1 cup	51	10.1	22
Buckwheat flour				
dark, sifted	1 cup	326	70.6	—
light, sifted	1 cup	340	77.9	—
Buckwheat Pancake Mix & Pan-cakes baked from mix				
See Pancakes				
Bulgur (parboiled wheat)				
dry, commercial, made from:				
club wheat	1 cup	628	139.1	—
hard red winter wheat	1 cup	602	128.7	—
white wheat	1 cup	553	121.1	—
canned, made from hard red	1 cup, unseasoned	227	47.3	809
winter wheat	1 cup, seasoned	246	44.3	621
Bullock's heart				
See Custard Apple				
Burger King				
Hamburgers				
Bacon Double Cheeseburger	1 sandwich	600	36	985
Cheeseburger	1 sandwich	360	35	705
Cheeseburger, Double	1 sandwich	520	35	865
Double Beef Whopper	1 sandwich	890	56	1,015
Double Beef Whopper with Cheese	1 sandwich	980	56	1,295
Hamburger	1 sandwich	310	35	560
Hamburger, Double	1 sandwich	430	35	585
Whopper	1 sandwich	670	56	975
Whopper with Cheese	1 sandwich	760	56	1,260
Whopper, Jr.	1 sandwich	370	35	545
Whopper, Jr. with Cheese	1 sandwich	410	35	685

Food	Quantity or Portion	Calories	Carbo-hydrates (grams)	Sodium (milli-grams)
Apple Pie	one pie	330	48	385
Chicken	1 sandwich	690	52	775
French Fries	regular size	210	25	230
Ham & Cheese	1 sandwich	550	43	1,550
Onion Rings	regular size	270	29	450
Shake, Chocolate	1 shake	340	57	280
Shake, Vanilla	1 shake	340	57	320
Veal Parmigiana	1 sandwich	580	46	805
Whaler	1 sandwich	540	57	745
Whaler with Cheese	1 sandwich	590	58	885
Burghul				
See Bulgur				
Butter, salted (a)				
regular type (1 brick or 4 sticks per lb)	1 stick (4 oz or ½ cup)	812	.5	1,119
	1 cup (2 sticks)	1,625	.9	2,240
	1 tbsp	102	.1	140
	1 tsp	34	trace	46
	1 pat (1″ sq)	36	trace	49
whipped type (6 sticks or two 8 oz containers per lb)	1 stick (2⅔ oz or ½ cup)	541	.3	746
	1 cup (2 sticks)	1,081	.6	1,490
	1 tbsp	67	trace	93
	1 tsp	23	trace	32
	pat (1″ sq)	27	trace	38
regular & whipped types	1 lb	3,248	1.8	4,477
Buttermilk				
fluid, cultured (made from skim milk)	1 qt	353	50.0	1,274
	1 cup	88	12.5	319
	1 lb	163	23.1	590
dried	1 lb pkg	1,755	226.8	2,300
	1 cup	464	60.0	608
	1 tbsp	25	3.3	33
Butternuts	1 lb in shell	399	5.3	—
	1 lb shelled	2,853	38.1	—

C

Cabbage
common varieties (Danish, domestic, pointed type)

raw	1 cup ground	36	8.1	30
	1 cup shredded coarsely or chopped	17	3.8	14
	1 cup shredded fine or chopped	22	4.9	18

(a) Unsalted butter contains approximately less than 10mg of sodium per 100g.

Food	Quantity or Portion	Calories	Carbo-hydrates (grams)	Sodium (milli-grams)
cooked (boiled until tender), drained				
shredded & cooked in small	1 cup	29	6.2	20
amount of water	1 lb	91	19.5	64
wedges, cooked in lg	1 cup	31	6.8	22
amount of water	1 lb	82	18.1	59
dehydrated	1 oz	87	20.9	54
Red, raw	1 cup shredded coarsely or sliced	22	4.8	18
	1 cup shredded fine or chopped	28	6.2	23
	1 lb	141	31.3	118
Savoy, raw	1 cup, shredded coarsely or sliced	17	3.2	15
	1 lb	109	20.9	100
Cabbage, Chinese (also called celery cabbage or petsai), raw	1 cup 1″ pieces	11	2.3	17
	1 lb	64	13.6	104
Cabbage, spoon (also called white mustard cabbage or pakchoy) (nonheading green leaf type, leaves & stems)				
raw	1 cup 1″ pieces	11	2.0	18
	1 lb	73	13.2	118
cooked (boiled), drained	1 cup 1″ pieces	24	4.1	31
	1 lb	64	10.9	82
Cabbage Salad				
See Coleslaw				
Cakes & Cupcakes, home baked				
Angelfood cake baked in tube	1 cake	1,926	431.0	2,026
pan, 9¾″ diam, 4″ high	1 piece, ½2 cake	161	36.1	170
	1 piece, ⅟₁₆ cake	121	27.1	127
cake 8½″ diam, 3½″ high	1 cake	1,270	284.1	33
	1 piece, ½2.cake	105	23.5	110
	1 piece ⅟₁₆ cake	81	18.1	85
Boston Cream Pie, 8″ diameter,	1 cake	2,492	411.7	1,535
3½″ high (2-layer cake with	1 piece, ⅛ cake	311	51.4	192
custard filling & powdered sugar topping)	1 piece, ½2 cake	208	34.4	128
Caramel				
without icing				
2 layers, 9″ diam, 3″ high	1 cake	3,326	464.0	2,635
2 layers, 8″ diam, 3″ high	1 cake	2,618	365.2	2,074
with caramel icing				
2 layers, 9″ diam, 3″ high	1 cake	4,779	745.3	3,178
	1 piece, ½2 cake	398	62.1	265
	1 piece, ⅟₁₆ cake	299	46.7	199
2 layers, 8″ diam, 3″ high	1 cake	3,790	591.0	2,520
	1 piece, ½2 cake	315	49.1	209
	1 piece, ⅟₁₆ cake	235	36.6	156

Food	Quantity or Portion	Calories	Carbo-hydrates (grams)	Sodium (milli-grams)
Chocolate (Devil's Food)				
without icing				
2 layers, 9" diam, 3" high	1 cake	3,257	462.8	2,617
2 layers, 8" diam, 3" high	1 cake	2,562	364.0	2,058
cake, sheet	1 piece, 3 × 3 × 2"	322	45.8	259
	1 piece, 2 × 2 × 2"	143	20.3	115
cupcake	2¾" diam	121	17.2	97
	2½" diam	92	13.0	74
with chocolate icing				
2 layers, 9" diam, 3" high	1 cake	4,402	665.7	2,804
	1 piece, ¹⁄₁₂ cake	365	55.2	233
	1 piece, ¹⁄₁₆ cake	277	41.9	176
2 layers, 8" diam, 3" high	1 cake	3,461	523.4	2,204
	1 piece, ¹⁄₁₂ cake	288	43.5	183
	1 piece, ¹⁄₁₆ cake	218	32.9	139
cake, sheet	1 piece, 3 × 3 × 2"	443	67.0	282
	1 piece, 2 × 2 × 2"	196	29.6	125
cupcake	2⅔" diam	162	24.6	103
	2½" diam	125	19.0	80
with uncooked white icing				
2 layers, 9" diam, 3" high	1 cake	4,354	698.6	2,761
	1 piece, ¹⁄₁₂ cake	362	58.0	229
	1 piece, ¹⁄₁₆ cake	273	43.8	173
2 layers, 8" diam, 3" high	1 cake	3,424	549.4	2,172
	1 piece, ¹⁄₁₂ cake	284	45.6	180
	1 piece, ¹⁄₁₆ cake	214	34.3	136
cake, sheet	1 piece 3 × 3 × 3"	435	69.9	270
	1 piece 2 × 2 × 2"	192	30.8	122
cupcake	2¾" diam	162	26.0	103
	2½" diam	122	19.5	77
Cottage Pudding, made with en-riched flour (8 × 8 × 1½)				
without sauce	1 cake	1,500	236.7	1,304
	1 piece, ⅙ cake	186	29.3	161
	1 piece, ⅛ cake	186	29.3	161
with chocolate sauce	1 piece, ⅙ cake, with 1⅓ tbsp sauce	315	56.1	231
	1 piece, ⅛ cake, with 1 tbsp sauce	235	42.0	172
with fruit sauce (strawberry)	1 piece, ⅙ cake, with 1⅓ tbsp sauce	274	45.5	219
	1 piece, ⅛ cake, with 1 tbsp sauce	204	33.9	163
Fruitcake, made with enriched flour				
Dark 1 lb loaf (7½ × 2 × 1½")	1 lb loaf	1,719	270.8	717
	1 slice, ¹⁄₃₀ loaf	57	9.0	24
Tube cake, 3 lb (7" diam, 2¼" high)	3 lb cake	5,158	812.5	2,150
	1 wedge, ¹⁄₃₂ cake	163	25.7	68
Light 1 lb loaf (7½ × 2 × 1½")	1 lb loaf	1,765	260.4	875
	1 slice, ¹⁄₃₀ loaf	58	8.6	29

Food	Quantity or Portion	Calories	Carbo-hydrates (grams)	Sodium (milli-grams)
Tube cake, 3 lb (7″ diam, 2¼″ high)	3 lb cake	5,294	781.2	2,627
	1 wedge, ⅟₃₂ cake	167	24.7	83
Gingerbread, made with enriched flour (9 × 9 × 2″)	1 cake	3,344	548.6	2,500
	1 piece, ⅑ cake	371	60.8	277
Plain Cake or Cupcake without icing				
cake, sheet (9 × 9 × 2″)	1 cake	2,828	434.3	2,331
	1 piece, ⅑ cake	313	48.1	258
cupcake	2¾″ diam	120	18.4	99
	2½″ diam	91	14.0	75
with chocolate icing				
cake, sheet (9 × 9 × 2″)	1 cake	4,081	658.7	2,540
	1 piece, ⅑ cake	453	73.1	282
cupcake	2¾″ diam	173	27.9	108
	2½″ diam	132	21.4	82
with boiled white icing				
cake, sheet (9 × 9 × 2″)	1 cake	3,619	635.3	2,693
	1 piece, ⅑ cake	401	70.5	299
cupcake	2¾″ diam	155	27.2	115
	2½″ diam	116	20.4	86
with uncooked white icing				
cake, sheet (9 × 9 × 2″)	1 cake	4,022	693.8	2,488
	1 piece, ⅑ cake	444	76.6	275
cupcake	2¾″ diam	172	29.8	107
	2½″ diam	128	22.2	79
Pound Cake, Old Fashioned loaf (8½ × 3½ × 3″)	1 loaf	2,431	241.6	565
	1 slice, ½″	142	14.1	33
Sponge Cake				
tube cake, 9¾″ diam, 4″ high	1 cake	2,346	427.4	1,319
	1 piece, ⅟₁₂ cake	196	35.7	110
	1 piece, ⅟₁₆ cake	146	26.5	82
tube cake, 8½″ diam, 3½″ high	1 cake	1,556	283.5	875
	1 piece, ⅟₁₂ cake	131	23.8	73
	1 piece, ⅟₁₆ cake	98	17.9	55
White Cake without icing				
cake, 2 layer, 9″ diam, 3″ high	1 cake	3,173	456.8	2,733
cake, 2 layer, 8″ diam, 3″ high	1 cake	2,490	358.6	2,145
White Cake with coconut icing				
cake, 2 layer, 9″ diam, 3″ high	1 cake	4,615	755.1	3,197
	1 piece, ⅟₁₂ cake	386	63.1	267
	1 piece, ⅟₁₆ cake	289	47.3	200
cake, 2 layer, 8" diam, 3" high	1 cake	3,625	593.0	2,511
	1 piece, ⅟₁₂ cake	301	49.2	208
	1 piece, ⅟₁₆ cake	226	37.0	157
White Cake with uncooked white icing				
cake, 2 layer, 9″ diam, 3″ high	1 cake	4,695	787.5	2,930
	1 piece, ⅟₁₂ cake	390	65.4	243
	1 piece ⅟₁₆ cake	293	49.1	183

Food	Quantity or Portion	Calories	Carbo-hydrates (grams)	Sodium (milli-grams)
cake, 2 layer, 8″ diam, 3″ high	1 cake	3,686	618.3	2,300
	1 piece, 1/12 cake	308	51.6	192
	1 piece, 1/16 cake	229	38.4	143
Yellow Cake, without icing				
cake, 2 layer, 9″ diam, 3″ high	1 cake	3,158	506.3	2,245
cake, 2 layer, 8″ diam, 3″ high	1 cake	2,476	396.9	1,760
Yellow Cake with caramel icing				
cake, 2 layer, 9″ diam, 3″ high	1 cake	4,692	794.4	2,929
	1 piece, 1/12 cake	391	66.2	244
	1 piece, 1/16 cake	293	49.7	183
cake, 2 layer, 8″ diam, 3″ high	1 cake	3,678	622.8	2,296
	1 piece, 1/12 cake	308	52.1	192
	1 piece, 1/16 cake	232	39.2	145
Yellow Cake with chocolate icing				
cake, 2 layer, 9″ diam, 3″ high	1 cake	4,391	726.6	2,502
	1 piece, 1/12 cake	365	60.4	208
	1 piece, 1/16 cake	274	45.3	156
cake, 2 layer, 8″ diam, 3″ high	1 cake	3,442	569.6	1,961
	1 piece, 1/12 cake	288	47.7	164
	1 piece, 1/16 cake	215	35.6	123
Cakes, Frozen (commercial)				
Devil's Food 1 lb 2 oz, with chocolate icing				
cake, 1 layer, 7½″ diam, 1¾″ high	1 cake	1,938	283.6	2,142
	1 piece, 1/6 cake	323	47.3	257
Devil's Food with whipped-cream filling, chocolate icing (1 lb 2 oz)				
cake, 2 layer, approx 7¼″ diam, 2″ high	1 cake	1,892	223.4	969
	1 piece, 1/6 cake	315	37.2	162
Cakes, Prepared & baked from mixes				
Angelfood, made with water, flavoring, tube cake, 9¾″ diam, 4⅜″ high	1 cake	1,645	377.2	927
	1 piece, 1/12 cake	137	31.5	77
	1 piece, 1/16 cake	104	23.8	58
Chocolate Malt, made with eggs & water, uniced 2-layer cake, 9″ diam, 2⅝″ high	1 cake	3,688	710.0	3,39
	1 piece, 1/12 cake	308	59.3	283
	1 piece, 1/16 cake	232	44.6	213
Coffee Cake, with enriched flour, made with egg & milk				
cake, 7¾ × 5⅝ × 1¼″	1 cake	1,385	225.3	1,853
	1 piece, ¼ cake	348	56.6	465
	1 piece, 1/6 cake	232	37.7	310
Cupcakes, made with egg & milk, without icing				
Yield from 11¾ oz of mix	12–16 cupcakes	1,400	223.2	1,812
	2¾″ diam	116	18.4	149
	2½″ diam	88	14.0	113

Food	Quantity or Portion	Calories	Carbo-hydrates (grams)	Sodium (milli-grams)
Cupcakes, made with egg & milk, with chocolate icing				
Yield from 11¾ oz mix with 6	12–16 cupcakes	2,041	337.4	1,910
oz (⅝ cup) cooked icing	2¾″ diam	172	28.4	161
	2½″ diam	129	21.3	121
Devil's Food, made with eggs & water with chocolate icing				
cake, 2 layers, 9″ diam, 2⅞″	1 cake	3,753	645.4	2,900
high or 8″ diam, 3¾″ high	1 piece, 1/12 cake	312	53.6	241
	1 piece, 1/16 cake	234	40.2	181
cupcake	2¾″ diam	156	26.8	121
	2½″ diam	119	20.4	92
Gingerbread, made with water				
cake, 8¼ × 8¼ × 1⅜″	1 cake	1,573	291.3	1,733
	1 piece, 1/9 cake	174	32.2	192
Honey Spice, made with eggs & water with caramel icing				
cake, 2 layers, 9″ diam, 2¾″	1 cake	4,347	752.1	3,026
high or 8″ diam, 3⅝″ high	1 piece, 1/12 cake	363	62.7	252
	1 piece, 1/16 cake	271	46.9	189
Marble, made with eggs & wa-ter, with boiled white icing				
cake, 2 layers, 9″ diam, 2¾″	1 cake	3,459	647.9	2,707
high or 8″ diam, 3½″ high	1 piece, 1/12 cake	288	53.9	225
	1 piece, 1/16 cake	215	40.3	168
White, made with egg whites & water, with chocolate icing				
cake, 2 layers, 9″ diam, 2⅔″	1 cake	4,001	715.9	2,588
high or 8″ diam, 3¾″ high	1 piece, 1/12 cake	333	59.7	216
	1 piece, 1/16 cake	249	44.6	161
Yellow, made with eggs & water, with chocolate icing				
cake, 9″ diam, 2⅞″ high or 8″	1 cake	3,734	638.2	2,515
diam. 3⅝″ high	1 piece, 1/12 cake	310	53.0	209
	1 piece, 1/16 cake	233	39.7	157
cupcake	2¾″ diam	155	26.5	104
	2½″ diam	118	20.2	79
Cake Icings, prepared from home recipes				
caramel	1 cup	1,224	260.1	282
chocolate	1 cup	1,034	185.4	168
coconut	1 cup	604	124.3	196
white, uncooked	1 cup	1,199	260.3	156
white, boiled	1 cup	297	75.5	134
Cake Icings, prepared from mixes				
chocolate fudge	1 cup	1,172	207.7	484
creamy fudge (contains nonfat dry milk)				
made with water	1 cup	831	182.8	568
made with water and table fat	1 cup	938	161.5	786

Food	Quantity or Portion	Calories	Carbo-hydrates (grams)	Sodium (milli-grams)
Cake Icings, ready to spread				
Betty Crocker Creamy Deluxe				
amaretto almond	½₂ container	170	26	90
chocolate	½₂ container	170	23	100
chocolate chip	½₂ container	160	26	80
chocolate chocolate chip	½₂ container	160	23	100
cream cheese	½₂ container	160	26	100
dark Dutch fudge	½₂ container	160	23	100
milk chocolate	½₂ container	160	24	100
vanilla	½₂ container	160	27	100
Duncan Hines Ready to Spread				
dark Dutch fudge	½₂ container	160	24	95
milk chocolate	½₂ container	160	24	85
vanilla	½₂ container	160	24	80
Pillsbury Frosting Supreme				
chocolate chip	½₂ container	150	27	70
chocolate fudge	½₂ container	160	24	80
cream cheese	½₂ container	160	26	115
double Dutch	½₂ container	140	22	45
lemon	½₂ container	160	26	80
milk chocolate	½₂ container	150	23	60
vanilla	½₂ container	160	26	75
Cake Mixes, brand names				
Betty Crocker Super Moist Pud-ding in the Mix				
apple cinnamon	½₂ cake	261	36	280
chocolate	½₂ cake	270	35	450
chocolate chip	½₂ cake	280	36	300
chocolate fudge	½₂ cake	250	35	450
devil's food	½₂ cake	270	35	430
yellow	½₂ cake	250	36	300
yellow, butter recipe	½₂ cake	260	37	350
Duncan Hines				
angel food, deluxe	½₂ cake	140	30	130
chocolate, deep	½₂ cake	280	33	375
chocolate chip	½₂ cake	260	34	265
chocolate, Swiss	½₂ cake	280	33	375
devil's food	½₂ cake	280	33	375
fudge marble	½₂ cake	260	36	285
golden	½₂ cake	270	36	270
lemon supreme	½₂ cake	260	36	285
strawberry supreme, deluxe	½₂ cake	260	36	285
yellow, deluxe	½₂ cake	270	36	270
Pillsbury Bundt				
Black Forest cherry	⅙₆ cake	240	38	310
Boston cream	⅙₆ cake	270	43	310
Pillsbury Plus Pudding in the Mix				
banana	½₂ cake	250	36	290
butter recipe	½₂ cake	240	36	345
carrot 'n spice	½₂ cake	260	36	330
chocolate chip cookie	½₂ mix	270	33	290
devil's food	½₂ cake	270	32	370

Food	Quantity or Portion	Calories	Carbo-hydrates (grams)	Sodium (milli-grams)
lemon	½ cake	220	31	260
yellow	½ cake	260	36	300
Pillsbury Streusel Swirl				
cinnamon	⅟₁₆ cake	260	36	200
lemon supreme	⅟₁₆ cake	270	39	335
Candied Fruits				
See Cherries, Citron, Ginger root,				
Grapefruit peel, Lemon peel,				
Orange peel, Pineapple				
Candy (use the following USDA				
amounts when actual values are				
not listed under Candy, brand				
names, below, or when container				
does not disclose nutritional val-				
ues)				
Butterscotch	1 oz	113	26.9	19
Candy Corn	1 cup pieces	728	179.2	424
	1 oz	103	25.4	60
Caramels				
plain or chocolate	1 oz	113	21.7	64
plain or chocolate with nuts	1 oz	121	20.0	58
Chocolate				
bittersweet	1 oz	135	13.3	1
semisweet	1 cup or 6 oz pkg tid-bits	862	96.9	3
	1 oz	144	16.2	1
sweet	1 oz	150	16.4	9
milk	1 oz, plain	147	16.1	27
	1 oz with almonds	151	14.5	23
	1 oz with peanuts	154	12.6	19
Chocolate coated almonds	1 cup single nuts	939	65.3	97
	1 oz single nuts or clusters	161	11.2	17
Chocolate coated coconut center	1 oz	124	20.4	56
Chocolate coated mints, round	1 lg, 2½" diam	144	28.4	65
	1 small, 1⅜" diam	45	8.9	20
	1 miniature, ¾" diam	10	1.9	4
Chocolate coated peanuts	1 cup single nuts	954	66.5	102
	1 oz, 8–10 single nuts or 2 clusters	159	11.1	17
Chocolate coated raisins	1 cup single raisins	808	134.0	122
	1 oz, 50 small or 18–28 lg raisins or clusters	120	20.0	18
Fudge				
Chocolate	1 oz	113	21.3	54
	1 cubic"	84	15.8	40
Chocolate with nuts	1 oz	121	19.6	48
	1 cubic"	89	14.5	36
Vanilla	1 oz	113	21.2	59
	1 cubic"	84	15.7	44

Food	Quantity or Portion	Calories	Carbo-hydrates (grams)	Sodium (milli-grams)
Vanilla with nuts	1 oz	120	19.5	53
	1 cubic"	89	14.4	39
Gumdrops, starch jelly pieces	1 oz	98	24.8	10
Hard candy	1 oz	109	27.6	9
Jellybeans (¾" long,½" wide)	1 cup (75 beans)	807	204.8	26
	1 oz	104	26.4	3
Marshmallows, plain	1 lg regular type (63 per lb)	23	5.8	3
	1 soft type (76 per lb)	19	4.8	2
	1 cup, miniature, not packed	147	37.0	18
	1 cup miniature, packed	179	45.0	22
	1 oz, all sizes	90	22.8	11
Mints, uncoated	1 oz	103	25.4	60
Peanut Bars	1 oz	146	13.4	3
Peanut Brittle (no added salt or soda)	1 oz	119	23.0	9
Sugar Coated:				
Almonds	1 cup	889	136.9	39
	1 oz	129	19.9	9
Chocolate Disks	1 cup	918	143.2	142
	1 oz	132	20.6	20
Candy, brand names				
Butterfinger	1 oz	130	19	50
Cadbury's				
Caramello	1 oz	140	18	55
dairy milk chocolate	1 oz	150	17	45
fruit and nut	1 oz	150	16	45
milk chocolate whole hazelnut bar	1 oz	150	16	45
roast almond	1 oz	150	15	40
Hershey's Milk Chocolate	1 oz	150	16	30
Hershey's Kisses	1 oz (6 kisses)	150	16	25
Milky Way	2 oz	260	43	140
M&M Peanut Chocolate Candy	1 oz	140	19	40
M&M Plain Chocolate Candy	1 oz	140	16	—
Reese's Peanut Butter Cup	2 med cups	250	23	170
Reese's Pieces	1 oz	140	17	—
Snickers	2 oz	270	33	150
Three Musketeers	2 oz	260	46	120
Cantaloupes				
See Muskmelons				
Cape Gooseberries				
See Ground-cherries				
Capicola or capacola				
See Sausage, cold cuts and luncheon meats				
Carambola, raw	1	20	4.5	1
Caraway Seed	1 tsp	29	1.05	trace
Cardamom, ground	1 tsp	6	1.37	trace

Food	Quantity or Portion	Calories	Carbo-hydrates (grams)	Sodium (milli-grams)
Carob Flour (Saint John's bread)	1 cup	252	113.0	—
	1 tbsp	14	6.5	—
Carrots				
raw, without tops	1 lb package	212	48.9	237
	1 carrot, 7½" long	30	7.0	34
	6–8 cut strips, 1 oz	12	2.7	13
	1 cup, grated or shredded	46	10.7	52
cooked (boiled), drained	1 cup sliced	48	11.0	51
	1 cup diced	45	10.3	48
	1 lb	141	32.2	150
canned, regular pack				
carrots & liquid	1 lb can	127	29.5	1,070
	1 cup	69	16.0	581
drained carrots	1 cup, sliced	47	10.4	366
	1 cup, diced	44	9.7	342
canned, special dietary pack (low sodium)				
carrots & liquid	1 lb can	100	22.7	177
	1 cup	54	12.3	96
drained carrots	1 cup	39	8.7	60
dehydrated	1 lb	1,547	367.9	1,216
	1 oz	97	23.0	76
Casaba melon				
See Muskmelons				
Cashew Nuts, roasted in oil	1 cup, whole kernels	785	41.0	21
	1 lb (200–240 lg, 260–320 med, or 350–500 small kernels)	2,545	132.9	68
	1 oz (14 lg, 18 med or 26 small kernels)	159	8.3	4
Cashews, brand names				
Planters				
Dry Roasted	1 oz	160	9	230
Fancy	1 oz	170	8	180
Catsup				
See Tomato Catsup				
Cauliflower				
raw, whole	1 head, 6–7" diam. 1.9 lb	232	44.7	112
raw, flowerbuds	1 cup, whole	27	5.2	13
	1 cup, sliced	23	4.4	11
	1 cup, chopped	31	6.0	15
cooked (boiled), drained	1 cup	28	5.1	11
	1 lb	100	18.6	41
frozen, cooked (boiled), drained	yield from 10 oz pkg	49	8.9	27
	yield from 1 lb frozen	77	14.2	43
	1 cup	32	5.9	18
Caviar, sturgeon				
granular	1 tbsp	42	.5	352
	1 oz	74	.9	624

Food	Quantity or Portion	Calories	Carbo-hydrates (grams)	Sodium (milli-grams)
pressed	1 tbsp	54	.8	—
	1 oz	90	1.4	—
Celery, green (Pascal type)				
raw	2 lb bunch	137	31.5	1,017
	8″ stalk, 1½″ wide	7	1.6	50
	1 small inner stalk, 5 × ¾″	9	2.0	63
	1 cup chopped or diced pieces	20	4.7	151
	1 lb	77	17.7	572
cooked	1 cup diced pieces	21	4.7	132
	1 lb (3 cups diced)	64	14.1	399
Celery Seed	1 tsp	8	0.83	3
Cereals, breakfast				
See Corn, Oats, Rice, Wheat, also Bran, Farina				
Cereals, breakfast, brand names				
Cream of Wheat	1 oz	100	22	80
General Mills				
Cheerios	1 oz	110	20	290
Cheerios, honey nut	1 oz	110	23	250
Cocoa Puffs	1 oz	110	25	200
Frosted Mini-Wheats	1 oz	100	24	5
Total—whole wheat	1 oz	110	23	280
Total—corn flakes	1 oz	110	24	310
Trix	1 oz	110	25	170
H-O				
Instant Oatmeal—Salt Free	½ cup	130	22	under 5
Instant Oatmeal—Raisin & Spices	½ cup	150	32	240
Instant Oatmeal—Regular	½ cup	110	18	230
Instant Oatmeal—Sweet & Mellow	½ cup	150	30	270
Quick Oats	½ cup	130	23	under 5
Kellogg's				
Apple Jacks	1 oz	110	26	125
All-Bran	1 oz	70	22	270
Bran Flakes	1 oz	90	23	220
Cocoa Crispies	1 oz	110	25	190
Corn flakes	1 oz	110	25	280
Corn Pops	1 oz	110	26	90
Crispix	1 oz	110	25	220
Frosted Flakes	1 oz	110	26	190
Fruit Loops	1 oz	140	33	290
Fruitful Bran	1 oz	120	30	230
Honey Smacks	1 oz	110	25	70
Lucky Charms	1 oz	110	24	180
Product 19	1 oz	110	24	320
Raisin Bran	1 oz	110	31	210
Rice Krispies	1 oz	110	25	280
Special K	1 oz	110	20	230

Food	Quantity or Portion	Calories	Carbo-hydrates (grams)	Sodium (milli-grams)
Nabisco				
100% Bran	1 oz	70	21	190
Shredded Wheat	1 oz	90	19	(a)
Shredded Wheat Spoon Size	1 oz	110	23	(a)
Shredded Wheat Toasted Wheat & Raisins	1 oz	100	23	0
Post				
Alpha-Bits	1 oz	110	24	80
Bran Flakes	1 oz	90	24	230
Fruit & Fiber with Dates, Raisins and Walnuts	1 oz	90	22	180
Fruit & Fiber—Harvest Medley	1 oz	90	23	190
Fruit & Fiber—Mountain Trail	1 oz	90	23	180
Fruit & Fiber—Tropical Fruit	1 oz	90	22	180
Grape-Nuts Flakes	1 oz	110	23	170
Honeycomb	1 oz	110	26	160
Horizon Trail Mix	1 oz	110	22	65
Raisin Bran	1 oz	90	23	160
Super Golden Crisp	1 oz	110	26	45
Quaker				
Cap'n Crunch	1 oz	120	24	220
Grits	1 oz	100	22	0
Instant Oatmeal—Apples & Cinnamon	1 packet	130	26	260
Instant Oatmeal—Bran & Raisins	1 packet	150	29	340
Instant Oatmeal—Cinnamon & Spice	1 packet	170	34	360
Instant Oatmeal—Raisins & Spice	1 packet	160	31	310
Life	1 oz	120	19	180
100% Natural	1 oz	140	17	15
100% Natural—Raisin & Date	1 oz	130	18	10
Puffed Rice	1 oz	50	13	0
Puffed Wheat	1 oz	50	11	0
Quick Oats	1 oz	110	18	0
Ralston				
Almond Delight	1 oz	110	23	200
Bran Chex	1 oz	90	23	300
Corn Chex	1 oz	110	25	310
Rice Chex	1 oz	110	25	280
Sun Flakes—Corn & Rice	1 oz	110	24	240
Sun Flakes—Wheat & Rice	1 oz	110	24	240
Wheatena	1 oz	120	21	0
Cervelat				
See Sausage, cold cuts & luncheon meats				
Chard, Swiss				
raw	1 lb	113	20.9	667

(a) Indicates miniscule amount.

Food	Quantity or Portion	Calories	Carbo-hydrates (grams)	Sodium (milli-grams)
cooked (boiled), drained	1 cup leaves & stalks	26	4.8	125
	1 cup leaves	32	5.8	151
	1 lb	82	15.0	390
Charlotte Russe with ladyfingers, whipped-cream filling	6 servings, 24 lady-fingers, 2 cups filling	1,959	299.5	295
	1 serving, ⅙ recipe	326	38.2	49
Cheeses, natural				
Blue or Roquefort type				
prepared cut pieces	4 oz pkg	416	2.3	—
	3 oz pkg	313	1.7	—
	1 cup crumbled, not packed	497	2.7	—
	1 cup crumbled, packed	916	5.0	—
	1 lb	1,669	9.1	—
	1 oz	104	.6	—
Brick				
prepackaged forms, cut piece	10 oz pkg	1,051	5.4	—
prepackaged forms, slices	8 oz pkg, 5 slices	840	4.3	—
	1 slice	167	.9	—
	1 lb	1,678	8.6	—
	1 oz	105	.5	—
Camembert (domestic)	4 oz pkg	338	2.0	—
	1 cup	736	4.4	—
	1 lb	1,356	8.2	—
	1 oz	85	.5	—
Cheddar (domestic type)				
prepackaged forms, cut piece	12 oz pkg	1,353	7.1	2,380
	10 oz pkg	1,130	6.0	1,988
	8 oz pkg	903	4.8	1,589
prepackaged forms, slices	6 oz pkg, 8 slices	677	3.6	1,190
	1 slice	84	.4	147
	10 oz pkg, 8 slices	1,130	6.0	1,988
	1 slice	139	.7	245
	8 oz pkg, 5 slices	903	4.8	1,589
	1 slice	179	.9	315
prepackaged form, squares	6 oz pkg (30 squares)	677	3.6	1,190
	1 cup	577	2.9	980
prepackaged form, shredded	1 cup, 4 oz pkg	450	2.4	791
	1 lb	1,805	9.5	3,175
	1 oz	113	.6	198
Cottage Cheese (dry curd with creaming mixture, 4.2% milk fat), lg or small curd	12 oz container	360	9.9	779
	1 cup, not packed, lg curd	239	6.5	515
	1 cup, not packed, small curd	223	6.1	481
	1 cup packed, lg or small curd	260	7.1	561
	1 lb	481	13.2	1,039
	1 oz	30	.8	65

Food	Quantity or Portion	Calories	Carbo-hydrates (grams)	Sodium (milli-grams)
Cottage Cheese (dry curd with-	12 oz container	292	9.2	986
out creaming mixture, 0.3%	1 cup, not packed	125	3.9	421
milk fat)	1 cup, packed	172	5.4	580
	1 lb	390	12.2	1,315
	1 oz	24	.8	82
Cream Cheese, regular	8 oz pkg	849	4.8	568
	3 oz pkg	318	1.8	213
	1 cup	868	4.9	580
	1 tbsp	52	.3	35
Cream Cheese, whipped	4 oz container	423	2.4	283
	1 cup	580	3.3	388
	1 tbsp	37	.2	25
Cream Cheese, regular &	1 lb	1,696	9.5	1,134
whipped	1 oz	106	.6	71
Limburger	7 oz pkg	683	4.4	—
	1 lb	1,565	10.0	—
	1 oz	98	.6	—
Parmesan				
cut pieces	5 oz wedge	558	4.1	1,042
	1 lb	1,783	13.2	3,329
	1 oz	111	.8	208
shredded	1 cup, not packed	338	2.4	629
	1 cup, packed	464	3.3	865
	1 tbsp	21	.2	39
	1 lb	1,914	13.6	3,565
	1 oz	120	.9	223
grated	1 cup, not packed	467	3.5	870
	1 cup, packed	654	4.9	1,218
	1 tbsp	23	.2	44
	1 lb	2,118	15.9	3,946
	1 oz	132	1.0	247
Swiss type, domestic				
cut pieces	12 oz pkg	1,258	5.8	2,414
	1 slice (2 × 2 × ¼″)	52	.2	99
slices	8 oz pkg, 7 slices	840	3.9	1,612
	1 slice	130	.6	249
	1 lb	1,678	7.7	3,221
	1 oz	105	.5	201
Cheese, pasteurized processed				
American				
prepackaged forms	32 oz (2 lb) pkg	3,356	17.2	10,304
	1 slice (2¾ × 2¼ × ¼″)	100	.5	307
	16 oz (1 lb) pkg	1,678	8.6	5,153
	1 slice (2½ × 1¾ × ¼″)	70	.4	216
	8 oz pkg	840	4.3	2,579
	1 slice (2⅛ × 1½ × ¼″)	48	.2	148
	1 cup, packed	944	4.8	2,897

Food	Quantity or Portion	Calories	Carbohydrates (grams)	Sodium (milligrams)
	1 cup diced, not packed	518	2.7	1,590
	1 cup shredded, not packed	418	2.1	1,284
slices	8 oz pkg, 8 sandwich-size slices	840	4.3	2,579
	6 oz pkg, 8 sandwich-size slices	629	3.2	1,931
	1 sandwich-size slice (3½ × 3⅜ × ⅛″)	105	.5	322
	1 sandwich-size slice (3½ × 3⅜ × 3/32″)	78	.4	239
	1 burger-size slice (3½ × 2¼ × ⅛″)	70	.4	216
	1 burger-size slice (3½ × 2¼ × 3/32″)	52	.3	159
Pimiento (American)				
prepackaged sandwich-size slices	8 oz pkg, 8 slices	842	4.1	—
	1 oz slice	105	.5	—
	12 oz pkg, 16 slices	1,261	6.1	—
	1 slice	78	.4	—
	1 lb	1,683	8.2	—
Swiss type				
prepackaged sandwich-size slices	8 oz pkg, 8 slices	806	3.6	2,649
	1 oz slice	101	.5	331
	12 oz pkg, 16 slices	1,207	5.4	3,968
	1 slice	75	.3	245
	1 lb	1,610	7.3	5,294
Cheese food, pasteurized process, American				
prepackaged forms	6 oz roll pkg	549	12.1	—
	1 slice, 1½″ diam, ¼″ thick, 1/18 roll	29	.6	—
	1 tbsp	45	1.0	—
	1 lb	1,465	32.2	—
Cheese souffle, homemade	1 souffle baked in 8″ sq pan or 7″ casserole	959	27.3	1,602
	1 portion, ¼ souffle	240	6.8	400
	1 cup (collapsed souffle)	207	5.9	346
	1 lb	980	28.1	1,651
	1 oz	62	1.8	103
Cheese spread, pasteurized process, American				
prepackaged form				
loaves (rectangular pieces)	32 oz (2 lb) pkg	2,612	74.4	14,739
	1 slice (2¾ × 2¼ × ¼″), 1/34 loaf	78	2.2	439
	16 oz (1 lb) pkg	1,308	37.2	7,371
	1 slice (2½ × 1¾ × ¼″), 1/24 loaf	55	1.6	309

CHEESE SPREAD

Food	Quantity or Portion	Calories	Carbo-hydrates (grams)	Sodium (milli-grams)
	8 oz pkg	654	18.6	3,689
	1 slice (2⅛ × 1½ × ¼"), 1/17 loaf	37	1.1	211
	1 cup, packed	734	20.9	4,144
	1 cup, diced, not packed	403	11.5	2,275
	1 cup, shredded, packed	325	9.3	1,836
	1 tbsp	40	1.1	228
packed in glass jars or pressurized can	5 oz jar	409	11.6	2,308
	4¾ oz can	389	11.1	2,194
	1 oz	82	2.3	461
Cheese Straws, 5" long, ⅜" wide, ⅜" high	10 pieces	272	20.7	433
Cherries				
raw				
sour red				
whole	1 qt container	410	101.0	14
	1 cup	60	14.7	2
	1 lb	237	58.4	8
without pits & stems	1 cup	90	22.2	3
	1 lb	263	64.9	9
sweet				
whole	1 cup	82	20.4	2
	10 cherries	47	11.7	1
	1 lb	286	71.0	8
without pits & stems	1 cup	102	25.2	3
	1 lb	318	78.9	9
canned, solids & liquid				
sour (tart) red, in water, pitted	1 lb can	195	48.5	9
	1 cup	105	26.1	5
sweet, in water, unsweetened,	1 lb can	200	49.7	4
light or dark cherries, unpitted	1 cup	119	29.6	2
sweet, in heavy syrup, unpitted	1 lb can	338	85.5	4
	1 cup	208	52.6	3
sweet, in heavy syrup, pitted	1 lb can	367	93.0	5
	1 cup	208	52.7	3
frozen, not thawed				
sour red, unsweetened	1 lb	249	60.8	9
sour red, sweetened with nutritive sweetener	1 lb	508	126.1	9
candied, whole	4 oz container	383	98.0	—
	10 cherries	119	30.3	—
	1 oz	96	24.6	—
Chervil, dried	1 tsp	1	0.3	trace
Chestnuts				
fresh	1 cup	189	40.9	6
	1 lb, 50 nuts (yields 2⅓ cups shelled nuts)	713	154.7	22
	10 nuts	141	30.7	4

Food	Quantity or Portion	Calories	Carbo-hydrates (grams)	Sodium (milli-grams)
shelled	1 cup	310	67.4	10
	1 lb (yield from approx 1¼ lb nuts in shell)	880	191.0	27
Chewing Gum (candy-coated	1 pkg, 12 pieces	63	19.0	—
pieces, approx ¾ × ½ × ¼")	1 piece	5	1.6	—
Chicken, cooked				
Broilers, ready-to-cook, broiled, meat only	7.1 oz, yield per 1 lb raw broiler	273	0	133
	12.5 oz, yield from 1¾ lb raw broiler (total cooked weight 1 lb 5 oz)	480	0	232
	1 lb	617	0	299
	1 portion (¼ lb)	154	0	75
Fryers, ready-to-cook, fried meat with skin & giblets	8 oz, yield 1 lb raw fryer	565	6.6	v
	1 lb 4 oz, yield from 2½ lb fryer (total cooked weight 1 lb 11 oz)	1,419	16.5	v
	1 lb	1,129	13.2	v
light meat without skin	1 lb	894	5.0	308
	1 portion (¼ lb)	224	1.2	77
	2 pieces each 2½ × 1⅞ × ¼"	99	.6	34
dark meat without skin	1 lb	998	6.8	399
	1 portion (¼ lb)	250	1.7	100
	4 pieces, each 1⅞ × 1 × ¼"	88	.6	35
cut-up parts from 2½ lb ready-to-cook fryer, fried	1 back piece	139	2.7	v
	½ breast	160	1.2	v
	1 drumstick	88	.4	v
	1 neck	127	2.0	v
	½ rib section	41	.8	v
	1 thigh	122	1.3	v
	1 wing	82	.8	v
Roasters, roasted meat, skin, giblets	8.4 oz, yield per 1 lb raw ready-to-cook roaster	576	0	v
	1 lb	1,098	0	v
light meat without skin	1 cup (not packed) chopped or diced	255	0	92
	ground	200	0	73
	1 lb	826	0	299
	1 portion (¼ lb)	207	0	75
	2 pieces each 2½ × 1⅞ × ¼"	91	0	33

Food	Quantity or Portion	Calories	Carbo-hydrates (grams)	Sodium (milli-grams)
dark meat without skin	1 cup (not packed)			
	chopped or diced	258	0	123
	ground	202	0	97
	1 lb	835	0	399
	1 portion (¼ lb)	209	0	100
	4 pieces each 1⅞ × 1 × ¼"	74	0	35
Hens and cocks, stewed meat, skin, giblets	8 oz, yield from 1 lb ready-to-cook	708	0	v
	1 lb	1,415	0	v
light meat without skin	1 cup (not packed)			
	chopped or diced	252	0	67
	ground	198	0	53
	1 lb	816	0	218
	1 portion (¼ lb)	204	0	55
	2 pieces each 2½ × 1⅞ × ¼"	90	0	24
dark meat without skin	1 cup (not packed)			
	chopped or diced	290	0	90
	ground	228	0	70
	1 lb	939	0	290
	1 portion (¼ lb)	235	0	73
	4 pieces each 1⅞ × 1 × ¼"	83	0	26
Chicken, canned, meat only, boned	5½ oz can	309	0	—
	1 cup	406	0	—
	1 lb	898	0	—
Chicken Frozen Dinners See Frozen Dinners				
Chicken Mix				
Chicken Helper	⅕ pkg without chicken	190	37	1,500
Chicken, potted See Sausage, cold cuts & luncheon meats				
Chicken a la king, home cooked	1 cup	468	12.3	760
	1 lb	866	22.7	1,406
Chicken fricassee, cooked, from home recipe	1 cup	386	7.7	370
	1 lb	730	14.5	699
Chicken Potpie				
home prepared, baked	1 lb	1,066	83.0	1,161
Chicken & noodles, home cooked	1 cup	367	25.7	600
	1 lb	694	48.5	1,134
Chickpeas or garbanzos, mature seeds, dry, raw	1 cup	720	122.0	52
	1 lb	1,633	276.7	118

Food	Quantity or Portion	Calories	Carbo-hydrates (grams)	Sodium (milli-grams)
Chicory, Witloof (also called French or Belgian endive), **raw**	1 5–7″ head	8	1.7	4
	1 cup, chopped ½″ pieces	14	2.9	6
	1 lb	68	14.5	32
Chili con carne, with beans, canned	15–15½ oz can	572	52.5	2,283
	1 cup	339	31.1	1,354
	1 lb	603	55.3	2,409
Chili Powder	1 tsp	7	1.1	31
Chili Sauce				
See Peppers & Tomatoes				
Chives, raw (chopped ⅛″ pieces)	1 tbsp	1	.2	—
	1 tsp	trace	.1	—
Chocolate				
bitter or baking	1 cup, grated	667	38.1	5
	1 oz	143	8.2	1
bittersweet				
See Candy				
Chocolate Syrup (or topping)				
thin type (chocolate flavored)	1 lb or 12 fl oz can	1,111	284.4	236
	1 cup	735	188.1	156
	1 fl oz or 2 tbsp	92	23.5	20
fudge type	1 lb or 12 fl oz can	1,497	244.9	404
	1 cup	990	162.0	267
	1 fl oz or 2 tbsp	124	20.3	33
Chop Suey, brand name				
La Choy				
Chop Suey Vegetables	½ cup, drained	10	2	320
Chow Mein, Chicken (without noodles)				
canned	1 lb can	172	32.2	1,315
	1 cup	95	17.8	725
Chow Mein, brand name				
La Choy				
Chicken Chow Mein	¾ cup	80	6	990
Fried Rice	¾ cup	190	40	960
Meatless Chow Mein	¾ cup	35	5	720
Cider, pasteurized				
See Apple juice				
Cinnamon, ground	1 tsp	6	1.84	1
Citron, candied	1 oz	89	22.7	82
Clams, raw, meat only				
soft	1 qt or 2 lbs (75 or less lg, 75–125 med, 125 or more small)	744	11.8	327
	1 pt or 1 lb (38 or less lg, 38–62 med, 62 or more small)	372	5.9	163

Food	Quantity or Portion	Calories	Carbo-hydrates (grams)	Sodium (milli-grams)
hard or round	1 qt or 2 lbs (28 or less chowders, 28–44 med, 44–62 cherry-stones, 62 or more little necks)	726	53.5	1,859
	1 pt or 1 lb (14 or less chowders, 14–22 med, 22–31 cherrystones, 31 or more little necks)	363	26.8	930
	4 cherrystones or 5 little necks	56	4.1	144
Clams, canned (type unspecified)				
clams & liquid	7⅛ to 8 oz can	114	6.2	—
	1 lb	236	12.7	—
drained clams	1 cup, chopped or minced	157	3.0	—
	1 lb	445	8.6	—
clam liquor, bouillon or nectar	8 fl oz bottle, or 1 cup	46	5.0	—
	1 fl oz	6	.6	—
Clam Fritters (2″ diam, 1¾″ thick)	1 fritter	124	12.4	—
Cloves, ground	1 tsp	7	1.29	5
Cocoa & chocolate-flavored instant beverage powders				
cocoa powder (instant) with non-fat dry milk	1 oz or 4 heaping tsp	102	20.1	149
cocoa powder (instant) without milk	1 oz or 4 heaping tsp	98	25.3	76
Cocoa, dry powder (a)				
plain	1 cup	228	44.3	5
	1 tbsp	14	2.8	trace
	1 oz (approx 5½ tbsp)	75	14.6	2
processed (with alkali)	1 cup	224	41.7	617
	1 tbsp	14	2.6	39
	1 oz (approx 5¼ tbsp)	74	13.7	203
Coconut Cream (liquid expressed from grated coconut meat)	1 cup	802	19.9	10
	1 tbsp	50	1.2	1
Coconut Meat				
fresh	1 coconut, about 3–5 cups, in shell	1,373	37.3	91
meat only	1 piece 2 × 2 × ½″	156	4.2	10
shredded or grated, spooned into cup	1 cup, not packed	277	7.5	18
	1 cup, packed	450	12.2	30
	1 lb	1,569	42.6	104
dried, unsweetened (desiccated)	1 lb	3,003	104.3	—
Coconut Milk (liquid expressed from mixture of grated coconut meat & coconut water)	1 cup	605	12.5	—
Coconut Water (liquid from coco-nuts)	1 cup	53	11.3	60

(a) Content may vary according to fat content of cocoa powder.

Food	Quantity or Portion	Calories	Carbo-hydrates (grams)	Sodium (milli-grams)
Cod				
cooked (broiled), with butter or margarine	1 steak, 5½" long, 4" wide, 1¼" thick, (un-cooked dimensions)	352	0	277
	1 fillet, 5" long, 2½" wide, ⅞" thick (un-cooked dimensions)	111	0	72
	1 lb	771	0	499
	1 oz	48	0	31
canned, drained	8½ oz can	204	0	—
	1 cup flaked	119	0	—
	1 lb	386	0	—
dehydrated, lightly salted	1 cup, shredded	158	0	3,402
	1 oz	106	0	2,296
dried, salted	1 piece 5½ × 1½ × ½"	104	0	—
	1 lb	590	0	—
	1 oz	37	0	—
Codfish Cakes				
See Fishcakes				
Coffee, instant, water-soluble				
dry powder, regular or freeze-dried	1 lb (makes approx 227 cups)	585	158.8	327
	1 oz (makes approx 14 cups)	37	9.9	20
	1 rounded tsp (makes 1 cup)	1	trace	1
beverage (prepared with 2 g dry powder, 1 rounded tsp, to 6 fl oz of water)	1 gal (approx 21 cups)	38	trace	38
	1 cup (6 fl oz)	2	trace	2
Cola or Coke				
See Beverages				
Coleslaw, made with				
French dressing	1 cup homemade	155	6.1	157
	1 cup commercial	114	9.1	322
mayonnaise	1 cup	173	5.8	144
salad dressing (mayonnaise type)	1 cup	119	8.5	149
Collards				
raw				
leaves without stems	20 oz container	255	42.5	—
	1 lb	204	34.0	—
leaves including stems	1 lb	181	32.7	195
cooked (boiled), drained (a)				
leaves without stems	1 cup	63	9.7	—
	1 lb	150	23.1	—
leaves including stems	1 cup	42	7.1	36
	1 lb	132	22.2	113

(a) Content may vary slightly according to the amount of water used for cooking.

Food	Quantity or Portion	Calories	Carbo-hydrates (grams)	Sodium (milli-grams)
frozen, chopped, cooked (boiled), drained	yield from 10 oz frozen (1½ cups)	75	14.0	40
	yield from 1 lb frozen (2⅓ cups)	120	22.4	64
	1 cup	51	9.5	27
	1 lb (yield from 1⅛ lb frozen)	136	25.4	73
Cookies				
Assorted (sandwich type, short-bread, sugar wafers, butter flavored, chocolate chip, co-conut bars, etc)	11 oz pkg (approx 36 cookies)	1,498	221.5	1,139
	1 lb (approx 52 cookies)	2,177	322.1	1,656
Brownies with nuts				
home baked	1 brownie, 3 × 1 × ⅞" or 1¾ × 1¾ × ⅞"	97	10.2	50
frozen, with chocolate icing, commercial	13 oz container	1,542	223.4	736
	1 brownie (¹⁄₁₅ con-tainer, 1½ × 1¾ × ⅞")	103	14.9	49
cookie mix, brand name				
Pillsbury Deluxe Fudge Brownie	1 prepared brownie	150	21	100
Betty Crocker Fudge Brownie	1 prepared brownie	130	21	95
Betty Crocker Brownie Supreme	1 prepared brownie	120	21	85
Duncan Hines Original Fudge Brownie	1 prepared brownie	160	22	105
Duncan Hines Peanut Butter Chocolate Brownie	1 prepared brownie	150	16	105
Butter, thin, rich (butter-flavored cookies)	8 oz pkg (approx 45 cookies)	1,037	160.9	949
	10 cookies	229	35.5	209
	1 lb (approx 90 cookies)	2,073	321.6	1,896
Chocolate Chip				
baked from home recipe, en-riched flour, each cookie 2⅓" diam	4 cookies	206	24.0	139
commercial type, each cookie 2¼" diam, ⅜" thick	14½ oz pkg, (approx 39 cookies)	1,936	286.5	1,648
	10 cookies	495	73.2	421
commercial type, each cookie 1¾" diam, ½" thick	7¾ oz pkg (approx 30 cookies)	1,036	153.3	882
	10 cookies	344	50.9	293
commercial type, each cookie 1¾" diam, ⅜" thick	15 oz pkg (approx 80 cookies)	2,002	296.2	1,704
	10 cookies	250	36.9	213
commercial cookies by the pound	1 lb	2,136	316.2	1,819

Food	Quantity or Portion	Calories	Carbo-hydrates (grams)	Sodium (milli-grams)
cookie mix, brand name Duncan Hines Chocolate Chip	2 cookies prepared as directed	130	20	85
Coconut Bars 2⅜ × 1⅝ × ⅜″ or 3 × 1¼ × 1¾″	10 cookies	445	57.5	133
	1 lb (approx 50 cookies)	2,241	289.9	671
Fig Bars (sq 1⅝ × ⅝″ or rectangular 1½ × 1¾ × ½″	1 lb pkg (approx 32 cookies)	1,624	342.0	1,143
	4 cookies	200	42.2	141
Gingersnaps (2″ diam, ¼″ thick)	1 lb pkg (approx 65 cookies)	1,905	362.0	2,590
	10 cookies	294	55.9	400
Ladyfingers (3¼ × 1⅜ × 1⅛″— dimensions before split lengthwise)	3 oz pkg (approx 8 ladyfingers split lengthwise)	306	54.8	60
	4 ladyfingers	158	28.4	31
	1 lb (approx 41 ladyfingers)	1,633	292.6	322
Macaroons (2¾″ diam, ¼″ thick)	11 oz pkg (approx 16 cookies)	1,482	206.2	106
	2 cookies	181	25.1	13
	1 lb (approx 24 cookies)	2,155	299.8	154
Marshmallow (plain cookie with marshmallow topping) coconut-coated, each cookie 2⅛″ diam, 1⅛″ thick	7½ oz pkg (approx 12 cookies)	871	154.0	445
	4 cookies	294	52.1	150
chocolate-coated, each cookie 1¾″ diam, ¾″ thick	8 oz pkg (approx 18 cookies)	928	164.1	474
	4 cookies	213	37.6	109
	1 lb	1,855	328.0	948
Molasses cookies	1 cookie, 3⅝″ diam, ¾″ thick	137	24.7	125
	1 lb (approx 14 cookies)	1,914	344.7	1,751
Oatmeal, with raisins, each cookie 2⅝″ diam, ¼″ thick	14 oz pkg (approx 30 cookies)	1,790	291.8	643
	4 cookies	235	38.2	84
	1 lb (approx 35 cookies)	2,046	333.4	735
Peanut (sandwich-type cookies or sugar wafers, with peanut filling) sandwich type	10 oz pkg (approx 23 cookies)	1,343	190.3	491
	4 cookies, each 1¾″ diam, ½″ thick	232	32.8	85

Food	Quantity or Portion	Calories	Carbo-hydrates (grams)	Sodium (milli-grams)
sugar wafer type	6¾ oz pkg containing 3 rectangular pieces, 8¾ × 2¾ × ⅜"; each marked for cutting into 10 cookies	903	128.0	330
	9 oz pkg (4 rectangular pieces	1,206	170.9	441
	10 cookies, each 1¾ × 1⅜ × ⅜"	331	46.9	121
sandwich type or sugar wafer	1 lb	2,146	303.9	785
Raisin (biscuit type)	7½ oz pkg (3 rectangular pieces, 10⅛ × 2¼ × ¼", each marked for cutting into 4 or 5 cookies)	807	172.1	111
	4 cookies, each 2¼ × 2½ × ¼"	269	57.4	37
	4 cookies, each 2¼ × 2 × ¼"	216	46.1	30
	1 lb	1,719	366.5	236
sandwich-type cookies (chocolate or vanilla)	1 lb pkg, approx 31 cookies	2,245	314.3	2,191
	4 oval cookies, each 3⅛ × 1¼ × ⅜" thick	297	41.6	290
	4 round cookies, each 1¾" diam, ⅜" thick	198	27.7	193
Shortbread cookies, 1⅝ × 1⅝ × ¼"	10¼ oz pkg, approx 40 cookies	1,449	189.4	175
	10 cookies	374	48.8	45
	1 lb	2,259	295.3	272
Sugar cookies, home baked, soft, thick with enriched flour, each cookie 2¼" diam, ¼" thick	10 cookies	355	54.4	254
Sugar Wafers				
cookie 3½ × 1 × ½"	13¼ oz pkg (approx 40 cookies)	1,824	276.0	711
	10 cookies	461	69.7	180
cookie 2½ × ¾ × ¼"	8½ oz pkg (approx 69 cookies)	1,169	176.9	455
	10 cookies	170	25.7	66
cookie 3½ × 1½ × ¼"	10 cookies	340	51.4	132
cookie 1¾ × 1½ × ¾"	10 cookies	437	66.1	170
	1 lb (approx 48 cookies)	2,200	332.9	857
Vanilla Wafers				
regular	12 oz pkg (approx 85 med or 113 small cookies)	1,571	253.0	857
	10 med cookes, each 1¾" diam, ¼" thick	185	29.8	101

Food	Quantity or Portion	Calories	Carbo-hydrates (grams)	Sodium (milli-grams)
	10 small cookies, each 1⅜″ diam, ¼″ thick	139	22.3	76
	1 cup crumbled	370	59.5	202
brown edge, 2¾″ diam, ¼″ thick, 78 per lb	10 oz pkg (approx 49 cookies)	1,312	211.3	716
	10 cookies	268	43.2	146
biscuit type, rectangular piece, 2¼ × 1½ × ¼,″ 96 per lb	11 oz pkg (approx 66 cookies)	1,441	232.1	786
	10 cookies	217	35.0	118
all types	1 lb	2,096	337.5	1,143
Cookies, prepared & baked from mixes				
Brownies, with enriched flour, made with incomplete mix, egg, water, nuts, rectangular piece, 3 × 1 × ⅞″ or sq piece 1¾ × 1¾ × ⅞″	1 brownie	86	12.6	33
Plain, with unenriched flour, made with egg, water, cookie 1⅝″ diam, ⅜″ thick	10 cookies	276	36.4	194
Cookie Dough, plain, chilled in roll				
unbaked, container, 18 oz, 10½″ long, 1¾″ diam	1 roll	2,290	299.9	2,530
baked cookie 2½″ diam, ¼″ thick, ¹⁄₄₀ roll	4 cookies	238	31.2	263
Cooking Oil				
See Oils				
Coriander Leaf, dried	1 tsp	2	0.31	1
Coriander Seed	1 tsp	5	0.99	1
Corn, sweet				
cooked (boiled), drained, white & yellow				
kernels, cut off cob before cooking	1 cup	137	31.0	trace
	1 lb	376	85.3	trace
kernels, cooked on cob	1 ear, 5″ long, 1¾″ diam	70	16.2	trace
	1 lb	227	52.4	trace
canned, regular pack				
cream style, white & yellow, not drained	17 oz can	395	96.4	1,138
	1 cup	210	51.2	604
	1 lb	372	90.7	1,070
whole kernel				
vacuum pack, yellow	7 oz can	164	40.6	467
	1 cup	174	43.1	496
	1 lb	376	93.0	1,070
wet pack, white & yellow				
corn & liquid	8¾ oz can	164	38.9	585
	1 cup	169	40.2	604
	1 lb	299	71.2	1,070
drained corn	1 cup	139	32.7	389
	1 lb	381	89.8	1,070

Food	Quantity or Portion	Calories	Carbo-hydrates (grams)	Sodium (milli-grams)
canned, special dietary pack (low sodium)				
cream style, white & yellow,	8¾ oz can	203	45.9	5
not drained	1 cup	210	47.4	5
	1 lb	372	83.9	9
whole kernel, wet pack, white & yellow				
corn & liquid	8¾ oz can	141	33.7	5
	1 cup	146	34.8	5
	1 lb	259	61.7	9
drained corn	1 cup	152	29.7	3
	1 lb	345	81.6	9
frozen				
kernels, cut off cob, cooked	1⅔ cups, yield from			
(boiled), drained	10 oz frozen	217	51.7	3
	2⅔ cups, yield from 1			
	lb frozen	348	82.7	4
	1 cup	130	31.0	2
	1 lb	358	85.3	5
kernels on cob, cooked	4 ears	474	109.0	5
(boiled), drained natural	1 ear	118	27.2	1
length ear, 5″ long	1 lb	235	53.9	2
Corn Flour	1 cup	431	89.9	1
	1 lb	1,669	348.4	5
Corn Fritters (2″ diam, 1½″ thick)	1 fritter	132	13.9	167
Corn Grits, degermed				
enriched or unenriched				
dry form	1 cup	579	125.0	2
	1 lb	1,642	354.3	5
cooked	1 cup	125	27.0	502
	1 lb	231	49.9	930
Corn Muffins				
See Muffins, Corn & Muffin mix, & Cornbread.				
Corn Oil				
See Oils				
Corn Products used mainly as ready-to-eat breakfast cereals				
Corn flakes				
plain, added sugar, salt, iron,	1 cup flakes	97	21.3	251
vitamins	1 cup crumbs	328	72.5	854
sugar coated, added salt, iron, vitamins	1 cup flakes	154	36.5	267
Corn, puffed				
plain, added sugar, salt, iron, vitamins	1 cup	80	16.2	233
presweetened, added salt,	1 cup without added			
iron, vitamins	flavor	114	26.9	90
	1 cup cocoa flavored	117	26.0	255
	1 cup fruit flavored	119	26.2	228

Food	Quantity or Portion	Calories	Carbo-hydrates (grams)	Sodium (milli-grams)
Corn, shredded, added sugar, salt, iron, thiamine, niacin	1 cup	97	21.7	269
Corn Pudding	1 recipe, approx 3 cups	770	96.2	3,226
	1 cup	255	31.9	1,068
Corn Syrup				
See Syrup, table blends				
Cornbread, home baked				
cornbread, southern style, made with whole-ground cornmeal	1 cornbread, 7½ × 7½ × 1½"	1,455	204.6	4,415
	1 piece, ⅑ of cornbread	161	22.7	490
corn pone, made with white whole-ground cornmeal, baked (9" diam, ¾" high)	1 whole pone	989	175.6	1,921
	1 sector, ⅛ of pone	122	21.7	238
spoonbread, made with white whole-ground cornmeal	1 cup	468	40.6	1,157
See also Muffins, Corn				
Cornbread, baked from mix				
See Muffin mix, corn & muffins & cornbread baked from mix				
Cornmeal, white or yellow				
whole ground, unbolted, dry	1 cup	433	89.9	1
bolted (nearly whole grain), dry	1 cup	442	90.9	1
degermed, enriched or unen-riched				
dry form	1 cup	502	108.2	1
cooked	1 cup	120	25.7	264
self-rising, whole ground	1 cup	465	96.3	1,849
self-rising, degermed	1 cup	491	106.2	1,946
Cornstarch, stirred	1 cup, lightly filled	463	112.1	trace
	1 tbsp, not packed	29	7.0	trace
Cottage Cheese & Cottage Cheese Dry Curd				
See Cheeses				
Cottage Pudding				
See Cakes				
Cottonseed Oil				
See Oils				
Cowpeas, including blackeye peas				
immature seeds				
raw	1 cup (blackeye peas)	184	31.6	3
	1 lb	576	98.9	9
cooked (boiled), drained	1 cup (blackeye peas)	178	29.9	2
	1 lb	490	82.1	5
canned, blackeye peas & liq-uid	1 lb can	318	56.2	1,070
	1 cup	179	31.6	602
frozen blackeye peas, cooked (boiled), drained	yield from 10 oz frozen blackeye peas, 1½ cups	338	61.1	101

Food	Quantity or Portion	Calories	Carbo-hydrates (grams)	Sodium (milli-grams)
	yield from 1 lb frozen blackeye peas, 2½ cups	546	98.7	164
	1 cup	221	40.0	66
	1 lb (yield from approx 17 oz frozen)	590	106.6	177
young pods with seeds				
raw	1 lb	200	43.1	18
cooked (boiled), drained	1 lb	154	31.8	14
mature seeds, dry				
raw	1 cup (blackeye peas)	583	104.9	60
	1 lb	1,556	279.9	159
cooked	1 cup	190	34.5	20
	1 lb	345	62.6	36
Crab, including blue, Dungeness, rock, king				
cooked (steamed)				
1 cup, not packed	pieces of crabmeat	144	.8	—
	flaked crabmeat	116	.6	—
1 cup, packed	pieces or flaked	195	1.1	—
pound	1 lb	422	2.3	—
Crab, canned				
drained contents from 6½ oz can (drained wt 4⅖ oz)	1 can, blue crab (claw or white)	126	1.4	1,250
drained contents from 7½ oz can (drained wt 6⅓ oz)	1 can, king crab	182	2.0	1,800
1 cup, not packed	claw	116	1.3	1,150
	white or king	136	1.5	1,350
1 cup, packed	claw, white or king	162	1.8	1,600
pound	1 lb	458	5.0	4,536
Crab, deviled	1 cup	451	31.9	2,081
	1 lb	853	60.3	3,933
Crab, Imperial	1 cup	323	8.6	1,602
	1 lb	667	17.7	3,302
Crackers				
Animal (approx 175 per lb)	2 oz pkg (approx 22 crackers)	245	45.5	173
	10 crackers	112	20.8	79
	1 lb	1,946	362.4	1,374
Butter				
whole				
round 1⅞″ diam, ³⁄₁₆″ thick (approx 138 per lb)	1 lb pkg	2,077	305.3	4,953
	10 crackers	151	22.2	360
rectangular, 2½″ long, 1⅜″ wide, ⅛″ thick (approx 120 per lb)	11½ oz pkg	1,493	219.4	3,560
	10 crackers	174	25.6	415
crumbed (finely crushed, spooned into cup without packing)	1 cup	336	53.8	874

Food	Quantity or Portion	Calories	Carbo-hydrates (grams)	Sodium (milli-grams)
Cheese				
whole, various shapes, up to 1⅞″ diam, ³⁄₁₆″ thick (145 per lb)	8½ oz pkg	1,154	145.6	2,504
	10 crackers	150	18.9	325
rectangular sticks 1⅝″ long, ¼″ thick (500 per lb)	11 oz pkg	1,494	188.4	3,242
	2¼ oz pkg	307	38.7	665
	10 crackers	44	5.5	95
round, 1⅞″ diam, ³⁄₁₆″ thick (approx 132 per lb)	8 oz pkg	1,087	137.1	2,359
	10 crackers	165	20.8	357
square, 1″, ⅛″ thick (approx 420 per lb)	10 oz pkg	1,360	171.5	2,951
	6¼ oz pkg	848	106.9	1,839
	2 oz pkg	273	34.4	592
	10 crackers	52	6.5	112
crumbed (finely crushed spooned into cup without packing)	1 cup	407	51.3	883
1 lb, whole or crumbed		2,173	274.0	4,713
Graham				
chocolate coated, each cracker 2½ × 2 × ¼″	1 lb	2,155	308.0	1,846
	1 cracker	62	8.8	53
plain, each cracker 2½″ sq	1 lb pkg	1,742	332.5	3,039
	2 crackers 2½″ sq	55	10.4	95
crumbed, finely crushed, spooned into cup	1 cup (approx 12 crackers), not packed	326	62.3	570
	1 cup (approx 15 crackers), packed	403	77.0	704
sugar honey	1 lb pkg	1,864	346.6	2,286
	2 crackers 2½″ sq	58	10.8	72
crumbed, finely crushed, spooned into cup	1 cup (approx 12 crackers), not packed	346	64.9	428
	1 cup (approx 15 crackers), packed	432	80.2	529
Saltines, 1⅞″ sq, ⅛″ thick (approx 160 per lb)				
whole	1 lb pkg	1,964	324.3	4,990
	7–7¼ oz pkg	875	144.4	2,222
	10 crackers	123	20.3	312
	4 cracker packet	48	8.0	123
crumbed, finely crushed, spooned into cup	1 cup (approx 24½ crackers), not packed	303	50.1	770
Sandwich type, cheese-peanut butter, 1⅝″ sq, ⅜″ thick, or round, 1⅝″ diam, ⅜″ thick	1½ oz packet—6 sandwiches	209	23.8	422
	1 oz packet, 4 sandwiches	139	15.9	281
	1 lb	2,227	254.5	4,500
Soda				
biscuit, 2⅜ × 2⅛ × ¼″ (approx 90 per lb)	3½ oz pkg	435	69.9	1,089
	10 biscuits	221	35.6	554
regular, 1⅞″ sq, ⅛″ thick (approx 160 per lb)	1 lb pkg	1,991	320.2	4,990
	10 crackers	125	20.1	312

Food	Quantity or Portion	Calories	Carbo-hydrates (grams)	Sodium (milli-grams)
soup or oyster, small, 530–650 per lb	1 lb pkg	1,991	320.2	4,990
	5 oz pkg	623	100.3	1,562
	1 cup	623	100.3	1,562
	10 crackers	33	5.3	83
crumbed (all types)	1 cup (14 biscuits, 25 sq crackers or 1½ cup oyster crackers)	307	49.4	770
Cranberries, raw	1 lb pkg	200	47.0	9
	1 cup, whole	44	10.3	2
	1 cup, chopped	51	11.9	2
Cranberry Juice Cocktail, bottled	1 pt bottle (16 fl oz)	329	83.5	5
(approx 33% cranberry juice,	1 qt bottle (32 fl oz)	658	167.0	10
sweetened with nutritive sweet-	1 cup	164	41.7	3
ener)	6 oz glass	124	31.4	2
	1 fl oz	21	5.2	trace
Cranberry Sauce, sweetened with	1 lb can	662	170.1	5
nutritive sweetener, canned,	1 cup	404	103.9	3
strained	½ oz packet	20	5.3	trace
	1 cup home prepared, unstrained	493	126.0	3
Cranberry-orange Relish, uncooked	1 cup	490	124.9	3
Cream, fluid				
See also, Non-Dairy Whipped Toppings				
half-and-half (cream & milk,	1 cup	324	11.1	111
11.7% fat)	1 tbsp	20	.7	7
light, coffee or table (20.6% fat)	1 cup	506	10.3	103
	1 tbsp	32	.6	6
whipping or light whipping	1 cup or approx 2 cups whipped	717	8.6	86
(31.3% fat)	1 tbsp	45	.5	5
heavy or heavy whipping (37.6%	1 cup or approx 2 cups whipped	838	7.4	76
fat)	1 tbsp	53	.5	5
Cream Substitute				
See Non-Dairy Cream				
Cream Puffs with custard filling	1 cream puff	303	26.7	108
(approx 3½″ diam, 2″ high)				
Cress, Garden				
raw	1 lb	145	24.9	64
cooked (boiled), drained (a)	1 cup	31	5.1	11
	1 lb	104	17.2	36
Croissants, Frozen, name brand				
Sara Lee All Butter				
Apple	1 croissant	170	19	(b)
Cheese	1 croissant	170	19	(b)

(a) Content may vary slightly according to the amount of water used and cooking time.

(b) Information not disclosed.

Food	Quantity or Portion	Calories	Carbo-hydrates (grams)	Sodium (milli-grams)
Cucumbers, raw				
not pared, whole				
lg, 2⅛″ diam, 8¼″ long (approx 1½ per lb)	1 cucumber	45	10.2	18
small, 1¾″ diam, 6⅜″ long (approx 2⅔ per lb)	1 cucumber	25	5.8	10
not pared, sliced (⅛″ slices)	1 cup	16	3.6	6
	6 large slices or 8 small slices	4	1.0	2
	1 lb whole or sliced	68	15.4	27
pared, whole	1 lg cucumber	39	9.0	17
	1 small cucumber	22	5.1	9
pared slices (⅛″ slices) or diced	1 cup	20	4.5	8
	6½ lg or 9 small slices	4	.9	2
	1 lb	64	14.5	27
Cucumber Pickles				
See Pickles				
Cumin Seed	1 tsp	8	0.93	4
Curry Powder	1 tsp	6	1.16	1
Cusk, steamed	1 lb	481	0	336
	1 oz	30	0	21
Custard, baked	1 cup	305	29.4	209
Custard, frozen				
See Ice Cream				

D

Food	Quantity or Portion	Calories	Carbo-hydrates (grams)	Sodium (milli-grams)
Dairy Substitutes				
See Non-Dairy Cream				
Dandelion Greens				
raw	1 lb	204	41.7	345
cooked (boiled), drained	1 cup greens, loosely packed (approx ½ cup pressed down)	35	6.7	46
	1 lb	150	29.0	200
Danish Pastry				
See Rolls & Buns				
Dates, moisturized or hydrated				
whole				
with pits	12 oz container	810	215.6	3
	10 dates	219	58.3	1
	1 lb	1,081	287.7	4
without pits	8 oz container	622	165.5	2
	10 oz container	778	207.0	3
	1 lb container	1,243	330.7	5
	10 dates	219	58.3	1
chopped	1 cup	488	129.8	2
Deviled Ham				
See Sausage, cold cuts & luncheon meats				

Food	Quantity or Portion	Calories	Carbo-hydrates (grams)	Sodium (milli-grams)
Dewberries				
See Blackberries				
Dill Seed	1 tsp	6	1.16	trace
Dill Weed	1 tsp	3	0.56	2
Dinners, Frozen				
See Frozen Dinners				
Doughnuts				
cake type, plain	2 oz doughnut, 3⅝" diam, 1¼" high	227	29.8	291
	1½ oz doughnut, 3 ¼" diam 1" high	164	21.6	210
	½ oz doughnut, 1½" diam, ¾" high	55	7.2	70
yeast leavened, plain, 3¾" diam, 1¼" high, approx 1½ oz	1 doughnut	176	16.0	99

E

Food	Quantity or Portion	Calories	Carbo-hydrates (grams)	Sodium (milli-grams)
Eclairs with custard filling & chocolate icing (5 × 2 × 1¾")	1 eclair	239	23.2	82
Eggs, chicken				
raw				
whole, fresh	1 ex lg	94	6.6	70
	1 lg	82	.5	61
	1 med	72	5.1	54
	1 cup (approx 4¼ ex lg, 4⅞ lg, or 5½ med eggs)	396	2.2	296
whites, fresh	egg white of 1 ex lg egg	19	.3	55
	egg white of 1 lg egg	17	.3	48
	egg white of 1 med egg	15	.2	42
	1 cup egg whites (egg whites of approx 6.4 ex lg, 7.4 lg, or 8.4 med eggs)	124	1.9	355
egg yolks	yolk of 1 ex lg egg	66	0.1	10
	yolk of 1 lg egg	59	0.1	9
	yolk of 1 med egg	52	0.1	8
	1 cup (egg yolks of approx 12.8 ex lg, 14.3 lg, or 16.2 med eggs)	846	1.5	126
cooked				
fried	1 ex lg egg	112	0.2	176
	1 lg egg	99	0.1	155
	1 med egg	86	0.1	135
hard cooked	1 ex lg egg	94	0.5	70
	1 lg egg	82	0.5	61

Food	Quantity or Portion	Calories	Carbo-hydrates (grams)	Sodium (milli-grams)
	1 med egg	72	0.4	54
	1 cup, chopped (approx 2.4 ex lg, 2.7 lg, or 3 med eggs)	222	1.2	166
omelet				
See scrambled				
poached	1 ex lg egg	94	0.5	154
	1 lg egg	82	0.5	136
	1 med egg	72	0.4	119
scrambled or omelet	1 ex lg egg	126	1.8	188
	1 lg egg	111	1.5	164
	1 med egg	97	1.3	144
	1 cup (yield from approx 3 ex lg, 3.4 lg, or 3.8 med eggs)	381	5.3	565
Eggs, duck, whole, fresh, raw	1 egg	134	0.5	86
	1 lb, approx 6½ eggs	866	3.2	553
Eggs, goose, whole, fresh, raw	1 egg	266	1.9	v
	1 lb (approx 3⅛ eggs)	839	5.9	v
Eggs, turkey, whole, fresh, raw	1 egg	135	1.3	v
	1 lb (approx 5.7 eggs)	771	7.7	v
Egg Substitute				
Egg Beaters	¼ cup	25	1	80
Eggplant, cooked (boiled), drained	1 cup, diced	38	8.2	2
	1 lb	86	18.6	5
Endive (curly endive & escarole)	1 cup, cut or broken into small pieces	10	2.1	7
	1 lb	91	18.6	64
Escarole, raw				
See Endive				

F

Food	Quantity or Portion	Calories	Carbo-hydrates (grams)	Sodium (milli-grams)
Farina, enriched or unenriched				
regular (about 15 min cooking time)	1 cup dry form	668	138.6	4
	1 cup cooked	103	21.3	353
quick cooking (about 2–5 min cooking time)	1 cup dry form	652	134.8	450
	1 cup cooked	105	21.8	466
instant cooking (about ½ min cooking time)	1 cup dry form	688	142.3	13
	1 cup cooked	135	27.9	461
Fast Food				
See individual restaurant names				
Fats, cooking (vegetable fat, mixed fat shortenings)	1 lb can	4,010	0	0
	48 oz (3 lb) can	12,361	0	0
	1 cup	1,768	0	0
	1 tbsp	111	0	0
Fennel Seed	1 tsp	7	1.05	2
Fenugreek Seed	1 tsp	12	2.16	2

Food	Quantity or Portion	Calories	Carbo-hydrates (grams)	Sodium (milli-grams)
Figs				
raw, whole	1 lg fig (approx 7 per lb)	52	13.2	1
	1 med fig (approx 9 per lb)	40	10.2	1
	1 small fig (approx 11 per lb)	32	8.1	1
canned, solids & liquid; whole style				
water pack, without artificial sweetener	1 lb can	218	56.2	9
	1 cup	119	30.8	5
	3 figs, 1¾ tbsp liquid	38	9.9	2
heavy syrup pack	17 oz can	405	105.1	10
	1 cup	218	56.5	5
	3 figs, 1¾ tbsp liquid	71	18.5	2
Filberts (hazelnuts)				
in shell	1 lb	1,323	34.9	4
	10 nuts	87	2.3	trace
shelled	1 cup whole	856	22.5	3
	1 cup, chopped	729	19.2	2
	1 tbsp, chopped	44	1.2	trace
	1 cup, ground	476	12.5	2
	1 lb	2,876	75.8	9
	1 oz (approx 20 nuts)	180	4.7	1
Fish				
See individual kinds: Cod, Flounder, etc.				
Fish Cakes				
fried				
regular size, 3″ diam × ⅝″ or 2½″ diam × ⅞″	1 cake	103	5.6	v
bite size, 1¼″ diam × ⅝″	1 cake	20	1.1	v
all sizes	1 lb	780	42.2	v
frozen				
regular size	1 cake	162	10.3	v
bite size	1 cake	32	2.1	v
all sizes	1 lb	1,225	78.0	v
Fish Flakes, canned, solids & liquid	7 oz can	220	0	v
	1 cup	183	0	v
	1 lb	503	0	v
Fish Frozen Dinners				
See Frozen Dinners				
Fish Loaf, cooked 8¾ × 4⅛ × 2½″	1 whole loaf	1,507	88.7	v
	1 slice 4⅛ × 2½ × 1″, ⅛ loaf	186	11.0	v
	1 lb	562	33.1	v
Fish Sticks, breaded, cooked, frozen, 4 × 1 × ½,″ wt 1 oz each	1 lb container, approx 16 fish sticks	800	29.5	v
	8 oz container, approx 8 fish sticks	400	14.8	v
	1 fish stick (1 oz)	50	1.8	v

Food	Quantity or Portion	Calories	Carbo-hydrates (grams)	Sodium (milli-grams)
Flounder, baked with butter or	1 fillet, 8¼ × 2¾ × ¼″	202	0	237
margarine	1 fillet, 6 × 2½ × ¼″	115	0	135
	1 lb	916	0	1,075
	1 oz	57	0	67
Flour				
See Corn, Rye, Soybean, Wheat				
Frankfurters				
See Sausage, cold cuts & lun-cheon meats				
French toast, Frozen, brand names				
Aunt Jemima	2 slices	170	26	560
Downeyflake	2 slices	270	30	380
Frostings				
See Cake Icings prepared from home recipes, also Cake Icings prepared from mixes				
Frozen Custard				
See Ice Cream				
Frozen Desserts, brand names				
Dole Fruit 'N Juice bars				
Pineapple	1 bar (2.5 fl oz)	70	17	5
Raspberry	1 bar (2.5 fl oz)	70	16	15
Strawberry	1 bar (2.5 fl oz)	70	16	5
Jell-O Gelatin Pops				
Raspberry	1 bar	35	8	5
Jell-O Pudding Pops				
Chocolate	1 bar	90	16	100
Chocolate Covered	1 bar	130	15	50
Chocolate-Vanilla Swirl	1 bar	90	16	80
Tuscan Pops (Low Fat Frozen Yogurt)				
Chocolate	1 bar	85	16	65
Strawberry	1 bar	130	16	60
Vanilla	1 bar	130	17	75
Tuscan Tofu				
Chocolate Coated Vanilla Almond	1 bar	170	16	60
Chocolate Covered Chocolate Royale	1 bar	170	17	70
Lemon Chiffon	1 bar	150	14	70
Weight Watchers Sandwich Bar	1 bar (2.75 fl oz)	130	28	75
Weight Watchers Treats				
Chocolate Mint	1 bar	100	19	75
Orange Vanilla	1 bar	100	19	75
Strawberry Vanilla	1 bar	100	19	75
Welch's Grape Juice Bar	1 bar (3 fl oz)	80	19	0
Frozen Dinners, brand name				
Buitoni				
Baked Shells	10.5 oz	320	55	(a)
Baked Ziti	10.5 oz	360	64	(a)

(a) Information not available.

Food	Quantity or Portion	Calories	Carbo-hydrates (grams)	Sodium (milli-grams)
Celentano				
Chicken Cutlets Parmigiana	9 oz	330	13	560
Eggplant Parmigiana	8 oz	330	22	405
Lasagne	8 oz	320	30	410
Lasagne Primavera	11 oz	300	17	500
Manicotti (without sauce)	7 oz	380	34	420
Stuffed Shells (without sauce)	6¼ oz	350	33	265
Le Menu				
Beef Sirloin Tips	11½ oz	390	26	825
Beef Stroganoff	10 oz	430	24	930
Breast of Chicken Parmigiana	11½ oz	400	27	895
Chicken Breast Florentine	12½ oz	480	40	850
Chicken Cordon Bleu	11 oz	440	50	865
Chicken a la King	10¼ oz	320	29	1,170
Chopped Sirloin of Beef	12¼ oz	410	28	1,080
Flounder fillet	10½ oz	350	27	1,125
Ham Steak	10 oz	320	35	1,510
Pepper steak	11½ oz	360	32	1,110
Sliced Turkey Breast	11¼ oz	470	36	1,165
Sweet & Sour Chicken	11¼ oz	460	45	720
Yankee Pot Roast	11 oz	360	29	830
Lean Cuisine (Stouffer)				
Cheese Cannelloni	9⅛ oz	270	24	950
Chicken a L'Orange	8 oz	280	27	460
Chicken Chow Mein with Rice	11¼ oz	250	36	1,160
Chicken Cacciatore	10⅞ oz	280	25	1040
Chicken & Vegetables	12¾ oz	260	28	1,250
Filet of Fish	12⅜ oz	270	17	770
Filet of Fish Florentine	9 oz	240	27	800
Filet of Fish Jardiniere	11¼ oz	280	18	810
Glazed Chicken	8½ oz	270	21	840
Linguini with Clam Sauce	9⅝ oz	260	32	860
Meatball Stew	10 oz	270	21	1,120
Oriental Beef	8⅝ oz	260	30	1,270
Stuffed Cabbage	10⅜ oz	210	19	830
Swanson				
Chopped Sirloin	11½ oz	350	29	930
Fried Chicken (Dark)	10¼ oz	610	55	1,390
Fried Chicken (White)	10¾ oz	660	64	1,610
Salisbury Steak	11 oz	460	44	1,050
Turkey	11½ oz	330	39	1,260
Veal Parmigiana	12¾ oz	470	49	1,120
Swanson Hungry Man				
Beef Pot Pie	16 oz	670	68	1,750
Boneless Chicken	17½ oz	670	60	1,640
Chicken Pot Pie	16 oz	700	64	1,670
Fried Chicken (White)	15¼ oz	880	73	2,120
Salisbury Steak	16½ oz	690	42	1,630
Turkey (Mostly White)	18½ oz	590	66	2,150
Turkey Pot Pie	16 oz	740	66	1,590
Veal Parmigiana	20 oz	640	62	2,010

Food	Quantity or Portion	Calories	Carbo-hydrates (grams)	Sodium (milli-grams)
Weight Watchers				
Breaded Chicken Patty Parmigiana	8 oz	290	13	(a)
Cheese Pizza	6 oz	350	37	670
Chicken Cacciatore	10 oz	290	30	(a)
Filet of Fish Au Gratin	9¼ oz	200	14	910
Imperial Chicken	9 oz	210	27	(a)
Italian Cheese Lasagna	12 oz	360	35	1,420
Lasagna	12 oz	360	40	(a)
Pepperoni Pizza	6¼ oz	370	38	(a)
Southern Fried Chicken Patty	6¾ oz	260	11	(a)
Spaghetti with Meat Sauce	10½ oz	280	36	(a)
Stuffed Turkey Breast	8½ oz	260	21	(a)
Veal Patty Parmigiana	8¹⁄₁₆	230	9	(a)
Ziti Macaroni	11¼ oz	290	32	(a)
Fruit Bars, Frozen				
See Frozen Desserts				
Fruit Cocktail, canned, solids & liquid				
water pack, without artificial	1 lb can	168	44.0	23
sweetener	1 cup	91	23.8	12
syrup pack, heavy	1 lb can	366	95.0	24
	1 cup	194	50.2	13
	1 lb	345	89.4	23
Fruit Rolls (Sunkist)				
All flavors (b)	½ oz	45	11	10
Fruit Salad, canned, solids & liquid				
water pack, without artificial	1 lb can	159	41.3	5
sweetener	1 cup	86	22.3	2
syrup pack, heavy	17 oz can	362	93.5	5
	1 cup	191	49.5	3
	1 lb	340	88.0	5

G

Food	Quantity or Portion	Calories	Carbo-hydrates (grams)	Sodium (milli-grams)
Garbanzos				
See Chickpeas				
Garlic, cloves, raw	1 clove	4	.9	1
Garlic Powder	1 tsp	9	0.05	1
Gelatin, dry				
envelope (wt 7 g or ¼ oz)	1 envelope	23	0	—
capsule (wt 10 grains)	1 capsule	2	0	—
Gelatin Dessert Powder and desserts made from powder				
powder	6 oz pkg	631	149.6	541
	3 oz pkg	315	74.8	270
	1 lb	1,683	399.2	1,422
	1 oz	105	24.9	90

(a) Information not disclosed.

(b) Content may vary slightly depending on flavor.

Food	Quantity or Portion	Calories	Carbo-hydrates (grams)	Sodium (milli-grams)
desserts (made with powder & water)				
plain	yield from 3 oz pkg (approx 2¼ cups)	315	74.8	270
	1 cup	142	33.8	122
with fruit added	yield from 3 oz pkg, 1 cup sliced bananas & 1 cup grapes (approx 3¼ cups)	563	137.8	286
	1 cup	161	39.4	82
Gelatin, brand names				
Jell-O				
all flavors (a)	½ cup	80	19	50
Sugar Free, all flavors (a)	½ cup	8	0	55
Royal Gelatin, all flavors (a)	½ cup	80	19	95
Gin				
See Beverages				
Ginger, ground	1 tsp	6	1.27	1
Ginger Ale				
See Beverages				
Gingerbread				
See Cakes				
Ginger Root, crystallized (candied)	1 lb	1,542	395.1	—
	1 oz	96	24.7	—
Ginger Root, fresh	1 lb	207	40.1	25
Gizzard				
chicken, cooked (simmered)	yield from 1 lb raw	497	2.4	192
	1 cup, chopped or diced pieces	215	1.0	83
	1 lb	671	3.2	259
turkey, cooked (simmered)	yield from 1 lb raw	659	3.7	171
	1 cup, chopped or diced pieces	284	1.6	74
	1 lb	889	5.0	231
Gluten Flour				
See Wheat Flour				
Goat Milk				
See Milk, Goat				
Goose, domesticated, cooked (roasted)				
total edible (flesh, skin, giblets)	8½ oz, yield from 1 lb ready-to-cook goose	1,022	0	—
	1 lb	1,932	0	—
meat only	1 lb (approx 13½ pieces)	1,057	0	562
	1 piece 3½ × 3 × ¼"	79	0	42
Gooseberries, raw	1 cup	59	14.6	2
Granadilla, purple (passion fruit), raw	1 fruit	16	3.9	5

(a) Content may vary slightly according to flavor.

Food	Quantity or Portion	Calories	Carbo-hydrates (grams)	Sodium (milli-grams)
Granola Bars, brand name				
Hershey New Trail				
Cocoa Cream	1 bar	200	21	60
Honey Graham	1 bar	200	21	55
Nature Valley Dandy Bar				
Chocolate Almond	1 bar	170	22	105
Milk Chocolate	1 bar	160	23	105
Peanut Butter	1 bar	160	21	120
Quaker Chewy Granola Bars				
Chunky Nut & Raisin	1 bar	130	17	95
Peanut Butter & Chocolate	1 bar	120	17	130
Raisin & Cinnamon	1 bar	130	19	100
Quaker Granola Dipps				
Caramel Nut	1 bar	140	20	95
Peanut Butter	1 bar	140	17	105
Raisin & Almond	1 bar	140	18	100
Rocky Road	1 bar	130	17	80
Ralston S'Mores				
Chocolate Fudge	1 bar	130	22	65
Peanut Butter & Chocolate Chip	1 bar	130	20	70
Grapefruit, fresh				
Pink & red, seeded	1 lg fruit, 4⅜" diam	137	35.6	3
	1 med fruit, 4³⁄₁₆" diam	116	30.1	3
	1 small fruit, 3¹⁵⁄₁₆" diam	103	26.8	3
	½ lg fruit	68	17.7	2
	½ med fruit	58	15.0	1
	½ small fruit	51	13.3	1
	1 cup sections	80	20.8	2
	1 cup sections with 2 tbsp juice	92	23.9	2
	1 cup cut-up fruit	70	18.2	2
Pink & red, seedless	1 lg fruit, 3¹⁵⁄₁₆" diam	109	28.4	3
	1 med fruit, 3¾" diam	98	25.6	2
	1 small fruit, 3⁹⁄₁₆" diam	82	21.3	2
	½ lg fruit	55	14.2	1
	½ med fruit	49	12.8	1
	½ small fruit	41	10.7	1
	1 cup sections	80	20.8	2
	1 cup sections with 2 tbsp juice	92	23.9	2
	1 cup cut-up fruit	70	18.2	2
White, seeded	1 lg fruit, 4⅜" diam	132	34.7	3
	1 med fruit, 4³⁄₁₆" diam	111	29.3	3
	1 small fruit, 3¹⁵⁄₁₆" diam	99	26.0	2
	½ lg fruit	66	17.4	2
	½ med fruit	56	14.7	1
	½ small fruit	49	13.0	1

Food	Quantity or Portion	Calories	Carbo-hydrates (grams)	Sodium (milli-grams)
	1 cup sections	82	21.6	2
	1 cup sections with 2 tbsp juice	94	24.8	2
	1 cup cut-up fruit	72	18.9	2
White, seedless	1 lg fruit, 3¹⁵⁄₁₆″ diam	102	26.5	3
	1 med fruit, 3¾″ diam	92	23.9	2
	1 small fruit, 3⁹⁄₁₆″ diam	77	19.9	2
	½ lg fruit	51	13.3	1
	½ med fruit	46	11.9	1
	½ small fruit	38	9.9	1
	1 cup sections	78	20.2	2
	1 cup sections with 2 tbsp juice	90	23.2	2
	1 cup cut-up fruit	68	17.7	2
Grapefruit, canned sections, solids & liquid				
water pack, without artificial sweetener	1 cup	73	18.5	10
syrup pack	1 lb can	318	80.7	5
	1 cup	178	45.2	3
Grapefruit Juice, fresh				
average of all varieties (a)	1 cup juice	96	22.6	2
	1 fruit 3⅜″ diam used for juice	80	19.0	2
from pink & red grapefruit, seeded	1 cup juice	93	22.4	2
from pink & red grapefruit, seed-less	1 cup juice	96	22.9	2
from white grapefruit, seeded	1 cup juice	98	23.4	2
from seedless (Marsh Seedless)	1 cup juice	93	22.1	2
Grapefruit juice, canned				
unsweetened	6 fl oz can	76	18.1	2
	1 cup	101	24.2	2
	1 fl oz	13	3.0	trace
sweetened with nutritive sweet-ener	6 fl oz can	99	23.9	2
	1 cup	133	32.0	3
	1 fl oz	17	4.0	trace
Grapefruit juice, frozen concen-trated unsweetened				
one can	6 fl oz can	300	71.6	8
diluted with 3 parts water by volume	1 qt	405	96.7	10
	1 cup	101	24.2	2
	6 oz glass	76	18.1	2

(a) Calorie and carbohydrate content varies slightly depending on the variety of grapefruit used. One whole grapefruit can yield from approx 6½ to 11 fl oz, depending on size of fruit. (8 fl oz = 1 cup)

Food	Quantity or Portion	Calories	Carbo-hydrates (grams)	Sodium (milli-grams)
sweetened with nutritive sweetener	6 fl oz can	350	85.2	6
diluted with 3 parts water by volume	1 qt	466	113.1	10
	1 cup	117	28.3	2
	6 oz glass	87	21.2	2
Grapefruit juice, dehydrated (crystals)				
dry form	1 oz	107	25.6	3
	1 lb (yields approx 1 gal juice)	1,715	409.6	45
prepared with water (1 lb crystals yields approx 1 gal juice)	1 cup	99	23.7	2
Grapefruit Juice & Orange Juice Blended				
canned				
unsweetened	6 fl oz can	80	18.7	2
	1 cup	106	24.9	2
	1 fl oz	13	3.1	trace
sweetened with nutritive sweetener	6 fl oz can	93	22.7	2
	1 cup	125	30.4	2
	1 fl oz	16	3.8	trace
frozen concentrated juice, unsweetened	6 fluid oz can (yields 24 oz, 3 cups, diluted juice)	330	77.9	4
diluted with 3 parts water by volume	1 qt	436	104.2	trace
	1 cup	109	26.0	trace
	6 fl oz glass	81	19.4	trace
Grapefruit Peel, candied	1 oz	90	22.9	—
Grapes, raw				
American type (slip skin) as Concord, Delaware, Niagara, Catawba, Scuppernong	10 grapes	18	4.1	1
	1 cup (approx 38 grapes)	70	15.9	3
	1 lb (approx 3 cups)	207	47.0	9
European type (adherent skin) as Thompson Seedless, Emperor, Flame Tokay, Ribier, Malaga, Muscat				
seedless types	10 grapes	34	8.7	2
	1 cup	107	27.7	5
seeded types	10 grapes	42	10.7	2
	1 cup	102	26.3	5
all varieties	1 lb	304	78.5	14
Grapes, canned				
Thompson Seedless, grapes & liquid				
water pack, without artificial sweetener	1 cup	125	33.3	10
	1 lb	231	61.7	18
syrup pack, heavy	8¾ oz can	191	49.6	10
	1 cup	197	51.2	10
	1 lb	349	90.7	18

Food	Quantity or Portion	Calories	Carbo-hydrates (grams)	Sodium (milli-grams)
Grape Juice				
canned or bottled	4 fl oz bottle	84	21.1	3
	24 fl oz bottle (1 pt, 8 fl oz)	502	126.2	15
	1 cup	167	42.0	5
	6 fl oz glass	125	31.5	4
frozen, concentrate, sweetened with nutritive sweetener				
undiluted	6 fl oz can (yields 24 fl oz, 3 cups, diluted juice)	395	100.0	6
	1 fl oz	66	16.7	1
diluted with 3 parts water by volume	1 qt	529	132.7	10
	1 cup	133	33.3	3
	6 fl oz glass	99	24.9	2
Grape Drink, canned (approx 30% grape juice)	32 fl oz (1 qt) can	540	138.0	10
	1 cup	135	34.5	3
	6 fl oz glass	101	25.8	2
	1 fl oz	17	4.3	trace
Gravy, brand names				
Franco-American				
Au Jus	2 oz	5	1	290
Beef	2 oz	25	3	310
Brown with Onions	2 oz	25	4	340
Chicken	2 oz	50	3	320
Turkey	2 oz	30	3	300
French's Gravy Mix				
Brown	¼ cup	20	4	250
Chicken	¼ cup	25	4	270
Turkey	¼ cup	25	4	290
Pillsbury Gravy Mix				
Brown	¼ cup	15	3	300
Home-Style	¼ cup	15	3	300
Griddlecakes				
See Pancakes				
Grits				
See Corn Grits & Cereals, Brand Names				
Ground-cherries (poha or Cape gooseberries), raw, without husks	1 cup	74	15.7	—
	1 lb	240	50.8	—

H

Food	Quantity or Portion	Calories	Carbo-hydrates (grams)	Sodium (milli-grams)
Haddock, fried (panfried or oven-fried)	12⅘ oz, yield from 1 lb raw fillets	597	21.0	641
	1 fillet, 6⅜ × 2½ × ⅝″ or 2¾ × 2½ × ⅞″	182	6.4	195
	1 lb	748	26.3	803
	1 oz	47	1.6	50

Food	Quantity or Portion	Calories	Carbo-hydrates (grams)	Sodium (milli-grams)
Halibut, Atlantic & Pacific, broiled with butter or margarine	12⅞ oz, the yield from 1 lb raw fillets	624	0	489
	1 fillet, 6½ × 2½ × ⅝″	214	0	168
	1 lb	776	0	608
	1 oz	48	0	38
Ham, fresh, cooked (baked or roasted)				
lean with fat	9.2 oz (yield from 1 lb raw with bone & skin)	980	0	148
	10.9 oz (yield from 1 lb raw without bone & skin)	1,152	0	173
	1 cup, not packed	524	0	79
	1 cup ground, not packed	411	0	62
	1 piece, ¼ lb	424	0	64
lean, trimmed of separable fat	6.8 oz (yield from 1 lb raw with bone & skin)	421	0	141
	8.1 oz (yield from 1 lb raw without bone & skin)	495	0	166
	1 cup, not packed, chopped or diced	304	0	102
	1 cup ground, not packed	239	0	80
	1 lb	984	0	330
	1 piece, ¼ lb	246	0	83
Ham (light cure, commercial), baked or roasted,				
lean with fat	11.3 oz (yield from 1 lb unbaked ham with bone & skin)	925	0	2,395
	13.1 oz (yield from 1 lb unbaked ham without bone & skin)	1,075	0	2,782
	1 lb	1,311	0	3,394
	1 piece, ¼ lb	328	0	848
lean, trimmed of separable fat	8.7 oz (yield from 1 lb unbaked with bone & skin)	460	0	2,227
	10.2 oz (yield from 1 lb unbaked without bone & skin)	539	0	2,610
	1 lb	848	0	4,110
	1 piece, ¼ lb	212	0	1,028
shoulder cuts (Boston butt & picnic)				
Boston butt, baked or roasted lean with fat	11 oz (yield from 1 lb unbaked with bone & skin)	1,030	0	2,556

Food	Quantity or Portion	Calories	Carbo-hydrates (grams)	Sodium (milli-grams)
	11.8 oz (yield from 1 lb unbaked without bone & skin)	1,109	0	2,753
	1 lb	1,497	0	3,720
	1 piece, ¼ lb	374	0	930
lean, trimmed of separable fat	9.1 oz (yield from 1 lb unbaked with bone & skin)	629	0	2,578
	9.8 oz (yield from 1 lb unbaked meat without bone & skin)	678	0	2,778
	1 lb	1,102	0	4,514
	1 piece, ¼ lb	275	0	1,128
Picnic, baked or roasted lean with fat	9.7 oz (yield from 1 lb unbaked meat with bone & skin)	888	0	2,205
	11.8 oz (yield from 1 lb unbaked meat with-out bone & skin)	1,085	0	2,696
	1 lb	1,465	0	3,637
	1 piece, ¼ lb	366	0	909
lean, trimmed of separable fat	6.8 oz (yield from 1 lb unbaked meat with bone & skin)	405	0	1,951
	8.3 oz (yield from 1 lb unbaked meat without bone & skin)	496	0	2,388
	1 lb	957	0	4,611
	1 piece, ¼ lb	239	0	1,153
Ham, canned	1 lb can	875	4.1	4,250
	3 lb can	2,627	12.2	12,754
	8 lb can	7,004	32.7	34,002
Hamburger **See Beef**				
Hamburger Mix, brand names Hamburger Helper				
Macaroni & Cheese	⅕ pkg without ham-burger	180	28	980
Beef Noodle	⅕ pkg without ham-burger	140	26	1,000
Lasagne	⅕ pkg without ham-burger	179	35	1,020
Ham Croquette (panfried), 1″ diam, 3″ long	1 croquette	163	7.6	222
	1 lb (approx 7 cro-quettes)	1,139	53.1	1,551
Hardee's (a)				
Apple Turnover	87g	282	37	—
Bacon Cheeseburger	244g	686	42	1,074

(a) Values shown are averages and may vary from restaurant to restaurant.

Food	Quantity or Portion	Calories	Carbo-hydrates (grams)	Sodium (milligrams)
Big Cookie	54g	278	33	258
Breakfast				
Bacon & Egg Biscuit	114g	405	30	823
Biscuit	82g	275	35	650
Cinnamon 'N' Raisin Biscuit	75g	276	30	346
Ham Biscuit	108g	349	37	1,415
Ham & Egg Biscuit	184g	458	37	1,585
Hash Rounds	71g	200	20	310
Sausage Biscuit	112g	413	34	864
Sausage & Egg Biscuit	162g	521	34	1,033
Steak & Egg biscuit	162g	527	41	973
Cheeseburger	116g	309	35	825
Chicken Fillet	192g	510	42	360
Fisherman's Fillet	196g	469	47	1,013
French Fries (small)	71g	239	28	121
French Fries (lg)	113g	381	44	192
Hamburger	110g	305	29	682
Big Deluxe	248g	546	48	1,083
Hot Dog	120g	346	26	744
Hot Ham 'N' Cheese	148g	376	37	1,067
Milkshake	326g	391	63	—
Mushroom 'N' Swiss	205g	512	46	1,051
Roast Beef Sandwich	143g	377	36	1,030
Big Roast Beef	167g	418	34	1,770
Shrimp Salad	336g	362	11	941
Turkey Club	194g	426	32	1,185
Hazelnuts				
See Filberts				
Headcheese				
See Sausage, cold cuts & luncheon meats				
Heart				
beef, lean, cooked (braised)	1 cup, chopped or diced	273	1.0	151
	1 lb	853	3.2	472
	1 oz	53	.2	2.9
calf, cooked (braised)	1 cup, chopped or diced	302	2.6	164
	1 lb	943	8.2	513
	1 oz	59	.5	32
chicken, cooked (simmered)	1 cup, chopped or diced	251	.1	100
	1 lb	785	.5	313
	1 oz	49	trace	20
hog, cooked (braised)	1 cup, chopped or diced	283	.4	94
	1 lb	885	1.4	295
	1 oz	55	.1	18
lamb, cooked (braised)	1 cup, chopped or diced	377	1.5	—
	1 lb	1,179	4.5	—
	1 oz	74	.3	—

Food	Quantity or Portion	Calories	Carbo-hydrates (grams)	Sodium (milli-grams)
turkey, cooked (simmered)	1 cup, chopped or diced	313	.3	88
	1 lb	980	.9	277
	1 oz	61	.1	7
Herring				
canned (fish & liquid)				
plain	15 oz can	884	0	v
	1 lb	943	0	v
in tomato sauce	1 herring (4¾ × 1⅛ × ⅝″) with 1 tbsp sauce	97	2.0	v
	1 lb	798	16.8	v
pickled				
Bismarck herring, 7″ long, 1 ½″ wide, ½″ thick	1 herring	112	0	v
marinated pieces	1 piece, 1¾ × ⅞ × ½″	33	0	v
	1 lb	1,012	0	v
	1 oz	63	0	v
smoked, kippered, canned (drained fish)	3¼ oz can	169	0	v
	8 oz can	411	0	v
	1 fillet, 7 × 2¼ × ¼″	137	0	v
	1 fillet, 4⅜ × 1¾ × ¼″	84	0	v
	1 fillet, 2⅜ × 1⅜ × ¼″	42	0	v
	1 lb	957	0	v
Hominy Grits, dry **See Corn Grits**				
Honey, strained or extracted	1 lb	1,379	373.3	23
	1 restaurant packet (½ oz, approx 2 tsp)	43	11.5	1
	1 cup	1,031	279.0	17
	1 tbsp	64	17.3	1
Honeydew Melon **See Muskmelons**				
Horseradish				
raw	1 lb	288	89.4	26
prepared	1 tbsp	6	1.4	14
	1 tsp	2	.5	5
Hyacinth beans, raw	1 cup young pods, cut	82	6.6	2
	1 lb mature seeds, dry	1,533	276.7	v

I

Food	Quantity or Portion	Calories	Carbo-hydrates (grams)	Sodium (milli-grams)
Ice Cream & frozen custard, plain (commercial) **See also Frozen Desserts**				
regular (approx 10% fat)				
hardened	½ gal	2,054	221.3	670
	1 qt or 8 slices	1,027	110.7	335

Food	Quantity or Portion	Calories	Carbo-hydrates (grams)	Sodium (milli-grams)
	1 slice, 4 fl oz	127	13.7	42
	1 cup, 8 fl oz	257	27.7	84
soft serve (frozen custard)	1 cup	334	36.0	109
rich (approx 16% fat), hardened	½ gal	2,637	213.8	392
	1 cup, 8 fl oz	329	26.6	49
Ice Cream, brand names				
Breyers				
Butter Almond	½ cup	179	15	125
Chocolate	½ cup	160	19	35
Coffee	½ cup	140	15	50
Natural Mint Chocolate Chip	½ cup	170	17	45
Natural Peach	½ cup	140	16	(a)
Natural Vanilla	½ cup	150	15	50
Vanilla Fudge Twirl	½ cup	160	18	45
Häagen-Dazs				
Chocolate	4 fl oz	283	25	(a)
Chocolate Chip	4 fl oz	309	25	(a)
Honey Vanilla	4 fl oz	267	24	(a)
Rum Raisin	4 fl oz	264	25	(a)
Strawberry	4 fl oz	267	25	(a)
Vanilla	4 fl oz	267	24	(a)
Ice Milk (5.1% fat)				
hardened	½ gal	1,593	234.8	713
	1 cup, 8 fl oz	199	29.3	89
soft serve	1 cup, 8 fl oz	266	39.2	119
Ices, water, lime	1 cup	247	62.9	trace
Icings				
See Cake Icings, homemade & Cake Icings, prepared from mixes				

J

Food	Quantity or Portion	Calories	Carbo-hydrates (grams)	Sodium (milli-grams)
Jams and Preserves, sweetened with regular amount of nutritive sweetener	10 oz glass or jar	772	198.8	34
	12 oz glass or jar	925	238.0	41
	½ oz restaurant packet, approx ⅔ tbsp	38	9.8	2
	1 tbsp	54	14.0	2
Jellies, sweetened with regular amount of nutritive sweetener	10 oz glass or jar	775	200.5	48
	½ oz restaurant packet, approx ¾ tbsp	38	9.9	2
	1 cup	819	211.8	51
	1 tbsp	49	12.7	3
Jello				
See Gelatin, brand names				

(a) Sodium content not disclosed.

Food	Quantity or Portion	Calories	Carbo-hydrates (grams)	Sodium (milli-grams)

K

Kale, leaves, without stems, mid-ribs
raw	1 lb	240	40.8	340
cooked (boiled), drained	1 cup	43	6.7	47
	1 lb	177	27.7	195

frozen (leaf kale)
cooked (boiled), drained
	yield from 10 oz frozen, 1⅔ cups	68	11.8	46
	yield from 1 lb frozen, 2⅔ cups	109	18.9	74
	1 cup	40	7.0	27
	1 lb, yield from 1.3 lb frozen kale	141	24.5	95

Kidney, beef, cooked (braised)
	1 cup, slices	353	1.1	354
	1 lb	1,143	3.6	1,148

Knockwurst
See Sausage, cold cuts & luncheon meats

Kohlrabi, thickened bulblike stems
raw, diced	1 cup	41	9.2	11
cooked (boiled), drained	1 cup, diced	40	8.7	10
	1 lb	109	24.0	27

Kumquats, raw, med size
	1 kumquat	12	3.2	1

L

Ladyfingers
See Cookies
Lamb, retail cuts
Leg of lamb, roasted
lean, with fat
	9.4 oz, (yield from 1 lb raw lamb with bone)	745	0	166
	11.2 oz (yield from 1 lb raw lamb without bone)	887	0	197
	1 cup, chopped or diced pieces (not packed)	391	0	87
	1 lb	1,266	0	281
	1 piece, ¼ lb (4 oz)	316	0	70

lean, trimmed of separable fat
	7.8 oz (yield from 1 lb raw lamb with bone)	411	0	186
	9.3 oz (yield from 1 lb raw lamb without bone)	491	0	186
	1 cup, chopped or diced pieces (not packed)	260	0	98

Food	Quantity or Portion	Calories	Carbo-hydrates (grams)	Sodium (milli-grams)
	1 lb	844	0	319
	1 piece, ¼ lb (4 oz)	211	0	80
Loin Chops, broiled				
lean with fat	10.1 oz (yield from 1 lb raw chops with bone)	1,023	0	154
	3.4 oz, 1 chop (3 per lb)	341	0	51
	2.5 oz, 1 chop (4 per lb)	255	0	38
	1 lb	1,628	0	245
lean, trimmed of separable fat	6.9 oz (yield from 1 lb raw chops with bone)	368	0	135
	2.3 oz, 1 chop (3 per lb)	122	0	45
	1.7 oz, 1 chop (4 per lb)	92	0	34
	1 lb	853	0	313
Rib Chops, broiled				
lean, with fat	9.5 oz (yield from 1 lb raw chops with bone)	1,091	0	132
	3.1 oz, 1 chop (3 per lb)	362	0	44
	2.4 oz, 1 chop (4 per lb)	273	0	33
	1 lb	1,846	0	223
lean, trimmed of separable fat	6 oz (yield from 1 lb raw chops with bone)	361	0	114
	2 oz, 1 chop (3 per lb)	120	0	38
	1.5 oz, 1 chop (4 per lb)	91	0	29
	1 lb	957	0	302
Shoulder of Lamb, roasted				
lean with fat	9.5 oz (yield from 1 lb raw lamb with bone)	913	0	144
	11.2 oz (yield from 1 lb raw lamb without bone)	1,075	0	169
	1 cup chopped or diced pieces (not packed)	473	0	74
	1 lb	1,533	0	241
	1 piece, ¼ lb (4 oz)	383	0	60
lean, trimmed of separable fat	7 oz (yield from 1 lb raw lamb with bone)	410	0	131
	8.3 oz (yield from 1 lb raw lamb without bone)	482	0	154
	1 cup chopped or diced (not packed)	287	0	92

Food	Quantity or Portion	Calories	Carbo-hydrates (grams)	Sodium (milli-grams)
	1 lb	930	0	298
	1 piece, ¼ lb (4 oz)	232	0	75
Lard	1 lb	1,091	0	0
	1 cup	1,849	0	0
	1 tbsp	117	0	0
Lasagna Frozen dinners				
See Frozen Dinners				
Lemons, raw				
whole fruit, peeled				
lg	1 lemon, 2⅜″ diam	29	8.7	2
	1 lemon, 2¼″ diam	24	7.1	2
med	1 lemon, 2⅛″ diam	20	6.0	1
slice	1 slice, ³⁄₁₆″ thick	2	.5	trace
wedges, with peel	¼ lg fruit	7	2.2	1
fruit, including peel				
lg	1 lemon, 2⅜″ diam	31	16.7	5
	1 lemon, 2¼″ diam	26	18.8	4
med	1 lemon, 2⅛″ diam	22	11.7	3
Lemon Juice, raw	1 cup	61	.5	2
	1 tbsp	4	1.2	trace
	yield from 1 lb lemons, ¾ cup	49	15.6	2
Lemon Juice, canned, unsweetened	6 fl oz can	42	.2	2
	1 cup	56	18.5	2
	1 tbsp	3	1.2	trace
	1 fl oz	7	2.3	trace
Lemon Juice, frozen, unsweetened	6 fl oz can	40	13.2	2
	1 tbsp	3	1.1	trace
Lemon Peel				
raw, grated (med grating)	1 tbsp	minimal	1.0	trace
	1 tsp	minimal	.4	trace
candied	1 oz	90	22.9	—
Lemonade concentrate, frozen				
undiluted	6 fl oz can (yields 1 qt (32 fl oz) lemonade)	427	111.9	4
diluted with 4⅓ parts water by	1 qt	427	111.9	4
volume	1 cup	107	28.3	1
	6 fl oz glass	81	21.1	1
Lentils, mature seeds, dry				
whole				
raw	1 cup	646	114.2	57
cooked	1 cup	212	38.6	—
split, without seedcoat, raw	1 cup	656	117.4	—
Lettuce, raw				
Butterhead varieties such as				
Boston types & Bibb				
whole, head approx 5″ diam	1 head	23	4.1	15
leaves	1 lg, 2 med or 3 small leaves	2	.4	1

Food	Quantity or Portion	Calories	Carbo-hydrates (grams)	Sodium (milli-grams)
	1 cup, chopped or shredded	8	1.4	5
	1 lb	64	11.3	41
Cos, or Romaine, such as Dark Green & White Paris	1 cup, chopped or shredded	10	1.9	5
	1 lb	82	15.9	41
Crisphead varieties such as Ice-berg, New York, Great Lakes strains				
whole, prepackaged trimmed head, approx 6″ diam, 1¼ lb	1 head	70	15.6	48
piece	1 piece, 5 × 4½″	3	.6	2
cut-up				
wedge, approx ¼ head	1 wedge	18	3.9	12
wedge, approx ⅛ head	1 wedge	12	2.6	8
	1 cup small chunks	10	2.2	7
	1 cup chopped or shredded	7	1.6	5
pound	1 lb	59	13.2	41
Looseleaf or bunching varieties such as Grand Rapids, Salad Bowl, Simpson	1 cup chopped or shredded pieces	10	1.9	5
	1 lb	82	15.9	41
Lima Beans				
See Beans, lima				
Limes, raw, pulp from fruit of 2″ diam	1 lime	19	6.4	1
Lime Juice, raw				
Juice	1 cup	64	22.1	2
	1 tbsp	4	1.4	trace
	juice from 1 lg lime, 2⅛″ diam	12	4.1	trace
	juice from 1 med lime, 2″ diam	10	3.5	trace
	juice from 1 small lime, 1⅞″ diam	9	3.0	trace
Lime juice, canned, unsweetened	1 cup	64	22.1	2
	1 tbsp	4	1.4	trace
	1 fl oz	8	2.8	trace
Limeade concentrate, frozen				
undiluted	6 fl oz can (yields 1 qt (32 fl oz) limeade)	408	107.9	trace
diluted with 4⅓ parts water by volume	1 qt	408	107.9	trace
	1 cup	102	27.0	trace
	6 fl oz glass	76	20.4	trace
Liver				
Beef liver, fried	1 slice 6½ × 2⅜,″ ap-prox 3 oz	195	4.5	156
	1 lb (approx 5⅓ slices)	1,039	24.0	835

Food	Quantity or Portion	Calories	Carbo-hydrates (grams)	Sodium (milli-grams)
Calves liver, fried	1 slice 6½ × 2⅜ × ⅜," approx 3 oz	222	3.4	100
	1 lb (approx 5⅓ slices)	1,184	18.1	535
Chicken liver, simmered	1 whole liver	41	.8	15
	1 cup chopped	231	4.3	85
	1 lb, approx 18 whole livers or 3¼ cups, chopped)	748	14.1	277
Hog liver, fried	1 slice 6½ × 2⅜ × ⅜," approx 3 oz	205	2.1	94
	1 lb (approx 5⅓ slices)	1,093	11.3	503
Lamb liver, broiled	1 slice 3½ × 2 × ⅜," approx 1.6 oz	117	1.3	38
	1 lb (approx 10 slices)	1,184	12.7	386
Turkey liver, simmered	1 liver from 20–25 lb turkey	212	3.8	67
	1 liver from 17 lb turkey	191	3.4	61
	1 liver from 12–13 lb turkey	131	2.3	41
	1 cup chopped	244	4.3	77
	1 lb	789	14.1	249
Liver Paste See Pate de Foie Gras				
Liver Sausage or liverwurst See Sausage, cold cuts & luncheon meats				
Lobster, Northern, cooked	1 cup ½" cubes	138	.4	305
	1 lb	431	1.4	953
Lobster Newburg	1 cup	485	12.8	573
Lobster salad (approx ½ cup of salad, wt 4 oz, with tomato wedges)	1 salad	286	6.0	322
Lobster Paste See Shrimp or Lobster Paste, canned				
Loganberries raw	1 cup	89	21.5	1
	1 lb	281	67.6	5
Loquats, raw	10 fruits	59	15.3	—
Luncheon Meat See Sausage, cold cuts & luncheon meats				
Lychees, raw	10 fruits	58	14.8	3

Food	Quantity or Portion	Calories	Carbo-hydrates (grams)	Sodium (milli-grams)

M

Macaroni, enriched or unenriched

dry form	1 lb pkg	1,674	341.1	9
	8 oz pkg	838	170.7	5
cooked, firm	yield from 1 lb dry form, 8.8 cups	1,674	341.1	9
	yield from 8 oz dry form, 4.4 cups	838	170.7	5
	1 cup, hot macaroni (cut lengths, elbows, shells)	192	39.1	1
	1 lb, yield from 6½ oz dry form	671	136.5	5
cooked, tender	yield from 1 lb dry form, 10.4 cups (hot) or 14 cups (cold)	1,674	341.1	9
	yield from 8 oz dry form, 5.3 cups (hot) or 7 cups (cold)	838	170.7	5
	1 cup, hot macaroni (cut lengths, elbows, shells)	155	32.2	1
	1 cup cold macaroni (cut lengths, elbows, shells)	117	24.2	1
	1 lb, yield from 5 oz dry form	503	104.3	5

Macaroni, (enriched) and Cheese

home baked	1 cup (served hot)	430	40.2	1,086
	1 lb	975	91.2	2,463
canned	15–15¼ oz can, approx 1¾ cups	409	46.0	1,307
	1 cup	228	25.7	730
	1 lb	431	48.5	1,379

Macaroni & Cheese, name brands

Kraft	¾ cup as prepared	290	34	530
Velveeta Shells and Cheese Dinner	¾ cup as prepared	260	32	720
Mace	1 tsp	8	0.08	1
Mackerel, Atlantic, broiled with butter or margarine	12⅞ oz (yield from 1 lb raw fillets)	861	0	—
	1 fillet, 8½ × 2½ × ½″	248	0	—
	1 lb	1,070	0	—
	1 oz	67	0	—
Mackerel, Pacific, canned, solids & liquid	15 oz can	765	0	—
	1 lb	816	0	—
Mackerel, salted	1 fillet 7¾ × 2½ × ½″	342	0	—
	1 lb	1,383	0	—
	1 oz	86	0	—

Food	Quantity or Portion	Calories	Carbo-hydrates (grams)	Sodium (milli-grams)
Malt, dry	1 oz	104	21.9	—
Malt Extract, dried	1 oz	104	25.3	23
Mamey (mammee apple), raw	1 fruit	446	109.3	181
Mandarin Oranges See Tangerines				
Mangos, raw	1 whole fruit	152	38.8	16
	1 cup diced or sliced	109	27.7	12
	1 lb	299	76.2	32
Margarine				
regular type (1 brick or 4 sticks per lb)	4 oz stick (approx ½ cup)	816	.5	1,119
	1 cup (approx ½ brick or 2 sticks)	1,634	.9	2,240
	1 tbsp (approx ⅛ stick)	102	.1	140
	1 tsp (approx ¹⁄₂₄ stick)	34	trace	46
	1 pat (1″ sq, ⅓″ high)	36	trace	49
soft type (two 8 oz containers per lb)	1 container (1 cup)	1,634	.9	2,240
	1 tbsp	102	.1	140
	1 tsp	34	trace	46
whipped type (6 sticks or two 8 oz containers per lb)	1 stick, 2⅔ oz (approx ½ cup)	544	.3	746
	1 cup (approx 2 sticks or ⅔ of 8 oz container)	1,087	.6	1,490
	1 tbsp (approx ⅛ stick)	68	trace	93
	1 tsp (approx ¹⁄₂₄ stick)	23	trace	32
	1 pat (1¼″ sq, ⅓″ high)	27	trace	38
regular, soft and whipped types	1 lb	3,266	1.8	4,477
Marjoram, dried	1 tsp	2	0.36	trace
Marmalade, citrus, sweetened with	12 oz jar	874	238.3	48
regular amount of nutritive	½ oz packet	36	9.8	2
sweetener	1 tbsp	51	14.0	3
	1 lb	1,166	318.0	64
Matai See Water Chestnut, Chinese				
Mayonnaise See Salad Dressings				
McDonald's				
Breakfast				
Egg McMuffin	138g	327	31	885
Hotcakes with Butter & Syrup	214g	500	93.9	1070
Scrambled Eggs	98g	180	2.5	205
Sausage	53g	206	.6	615
English Muffin with Butter	63g	186	29.5	318
Hash Brown Potatoes	55g	125	14	325

Food	Quantity or Portion	Calories	Carbo-hydrates (grams)	Sodium (milli-grams)
Burgers				
Hamburger	102g	255	29.5	520
Cheeseburger	115g	307	19.8	767
Quarter Pounder	166g	424	32.7	735
Quarter Pounder with Cheese	194g	524	32.2	1,236
Big Mac	204g	563	40.6	1,010
Chicken McNuggets	6 pieces	314	15.4	525
Filet-O-Fish	139g	432	37.4	781
Fries, regular	68g	220	26.1	109
Shakes				
Chocolate	291g	383	65.5	300
Strawberry	290g	362	62.1	207
Vanilla	291g	352	59.6	201
Sundaes				
Caramel	165g	328	52.5	195
Hot Fudge	164g	310	46.2	175
Strawberry	164g	289	46.1	96.4
Cake Cones	115g	185	30.2	109
Pies				
Apple	85g	253	29.3	398
Cherry	88g	260	32.1	427
Cookies				
Chocolaty Chip	69g	342	44.8	313
McDonaldland	67g	308	48.7	358
Meat				
See Beef, Lamb, Pork, Veal				
Meat Loaf				
See Sausage, cold cuts & luncheon meats				
Melba Toast, name brand				
Old London				
Pumpernickel	½ oz (about 3 slices)	50	10	170
Sesame	½ oz (about 3 slices)	60	9	160
Wheat or Rye	½ oz (about 3 slices)	50	10	130
Melons				
See Muskmelons & Watermelon				
Milk, buttermilk				
See Buttermilk				
Milk, canned				
evaporated (unsweetened)	1 cup	345	24.4	297
	1 fl oz	43	3.1	37
condensed (sweetened)	1 cup	982	166.2	343
	1 fl oz	123	20.7	43
Milk, chocolate drink, fluid, commercial (approx 90% milk)				
made with skim milk (2% butterfat added)	1 qt	760	109.0	460
	1 cup	190	27.3	115
made with whole 3.5% fat milk	1 qt	850	110.0	470
	1 cup	213	27.5	118

Food	Quantity or Portion	Calories	Carbo-hydrates (grams)	Sodium (milli-grams)
Milk, chocolate beverages, home-made				
hot chocolate	1 cup	238	26.0	120
hot cocoa	1 cup	243	27.3	128
Milk, cow, fluid (pasteurized or raw)				
whole, 3.5% fat	1 qt	634	47.8	488
	1 cup	159	12.0	122
skim	1 qt	353	50.0	.4
	1 cup	88	12.5	127
low fat with 2% nonfat milk solids	1 qt	581	59.0	600
added	1 cup	145	14.8	150
half-and-half (cream & milk) See Cream				
Milk, dry				
whole				
regular	1 cup	643	48.9	518
regular & instant	1 lb	2,277	173.3	1,837
nonfat, regular	1 cup dry	436	62.8	638
nonfat, instant (one 3.2 oz enve-lope (approx 1⅓ cups dry) added to 3¾ cups water makes 4 cups (1 qt) milk)	1 envelope	327	47.0	479
Milk prepared from brand name powder as directed:				
Alba brand	1 cup (8 fl oz)	80	12	190
	1 qt (32 fl oz)	320	48	760
Carnation brand	1 cup (8 fl oz)	80	12	125
	1 qt (32 fl oz)	320	48	500
Milk, goat, fluid	1 qt	654	44.9	332
	1 cup	163	11.2	83
Milk, human, U.S. samples	1 fl oz	24	2.9	5
Milk, malted				
dry powder	1 oz or approx 3 heaping tsp	116	20.1	125
beverage, from powder & whole milk	1 cup	244	27.5	214
Milk, reindeer	1 cup	580	10.2	389
Mixed Vegetables; frozen See Vegetables, mixed, frozen				
Molasses, cane				
first extraction or light	12 fl oz bottle	1,242	320.5	74
	1 cup	827	213.2	49
	1 tbsp	50	13.0	3
	1 fl oz	103	26.7	6
second extraction or med	12 fl oz bottle	1,444	295.8	182
	1 cup	761	196.8	121
	1 tbsp	46	12.0	7
	1 fl oz	95	24.6	15
third extraction or blackstrap	12 oz bottle	1,050	271.2	473
	1 cup	699	180.4	315

Food	Quantity or Portion	Calories	Carbo-hydrates (grams)	Sodium (milli-grams)
	1 tbsp	43	11.0	19
	1 fl oz	87	22.6	39
Mortadella				
See Sausage, cold cuts & luncheon meats				
Muffins, home baked				
plain, made with enriched or unenriched flour	1 muffin (3″ diam at top, 2″ diam at bottom, 1½″ high; yield from approx 3 tbsp batter)	118	16.9	176
	1 lb	1,334	191.9	2,000
blueberry	1 muffin (2⅜″ diam at top, 2″ diam at bottom, 1½″ high; yield from approx 3 tbsp batter)	112	16.8	253
	1 lb	1,275	190.1	2,867
bran	1 muffin (2⅝″ diam at top, 2″ diam at bottom, 1⅜″ high; yield from approx ¼ cup batter)	104	17.2	179
	1 lb	1,184	195.5	2,032
corn, made with enriched degermed cornmeal	1 muffin (2⅜″ diam at top, 2″ diam at bottom, 1½″ high; yield from approx ¼ cup batter)	126	19.2	192
	1 lb	1,424	218.2	2,182
corn, made with whole-ground cornmeal	1 muffin (2⅜″ diam at top, 2″ diam at bottom, 1½″ high; yield from approx ¼ cup batter)	115	17.0	198
	1 lb	1,306	192.8	2,245
Muffin mix (corn) & muffins & cornbread baked from mix				
mix, dry form, with enriched flour	1 cup, not packed	542	93.3	858
	1 cup, packed	709	122.1	1,122
muffins & cornbread, made from mix with egg & milk				
muffin, 2⅜″ diam at top, 2″ diam at bottom, 1½″ high	1 muffin (yield from approx ¼ cup batter)	130	20.0	192
cornbread, 7½ × 7½ × 1⅜″	1 whole cornbread, yield from 12 oz mix	1,620	250.0	2,395
	1 piece, 2½ × 2½ × 1⅜″, ⅑ cornbread	178	27.5	263
	1 cube, 1 cubic″	21	3.3	31
	1 lb	1,470	1,093	2,173
Mushrooms				
agaricus campestris, cultivated commercially, raw	1 cup sliced, chopped or diced	20	3.1	11
	1 lb	127	20.0	68

Food	Quantity or Portion	Calories	Carbo-hydrates (grams)	Sodium (milli-grams)
other edible species, raw	1 cup sliced, chopped, or diced	25	4.6	7
	1 lb	159	29.5	45
Muskmelons, raw				
cantaloupes with orange-colored flesh	1 whole 2⅓ lb melon, 5″ diam	159	39.8	64
	½ melon	82	20.4	33
	1 cup cubed or diced pieces, melon balls (approx 20 per cup)	48	12.0	19
	1 lb pieces	136	34.0	54
casaba (golden beauty)	1 whole 6 lb melon, 6½″ diam, 7¾″ long	367	88.5	163
	1 wedge, 7¾″ long, 2″ wide at center, ¹⁄₁₀ melon	38	9.1	17
	1 cup cubed or diced pieces, melon balls (approx 20 per cup)	46	11.1	20
	1 lb pieces	122	29.5	54
honeydew	1 whole 5¼ lb melon, 6½″ diam, 7″ long	495	115.5	180
	1 wedge, 7″ long, 2″ wide at center, ¹⁄₁₀ melon	49	11.5	18
	1 cup cubed or diced pieces, melon balls (approx 20 per cup)	56	13.1	20
	1 lb pieces	150	34.9	54
Muskmelons, frozen				
melon balls (cantaloupe & honeydew) in syrup, not thawed	12 oz container	211	53.4	31
	1 cup	143	36.1	21
	1 lb	281	71.2	41
Mustard, prepared				
brown	1 cup	228	13.3	3,268
	1 tsp, individual serving pouch or cup	5	.3	65
yellow	1 cup	188	16.0	3,130
	1 tsp, individual serving pouch or cup	4	.3	63
Mustard Greens				
raw	1 lb	141	25.4	145
cooked (boiled), drained	1 cup leaves, without stems, midribs	32	5.6	25
	1 lb	104	18.1	82
frozen, chopped, cooked (boiled) & drained	1.4 cups, yield from 10 oz frozen	42	6.6	21
	2¼ cups, yield from 1 lb frozen	68	10.5	34

Food	Quantity or Portion	Calories	Carbo-hydrates (grams)	Sodium (milli-grams)
	1 cup	30	4.7	15
	1 lb (yield from 1⅓ lb frozen)	91	14.1	45
Mustard Seed, yellow	1 tsp	15	1.15	trace
Mustard Spinach (tendergreen)				
raw	1 lb	100	17.7	—
cooked (boiled), drained	1 cup	29	5.0	—
	1 lb	73	12.7	—

N

Food	Quantity or Portion	Calories	Carbo-hydrates (grams)	Sodium (milli-grams)
Nectarines, raw, 2½″ diam	1 nectarine	88	23.6	8
New Zealand Spinach				
raw	1 lb	86	14.1	721
cooked (boiled), drained	1 cup	23	3.8	166
	1 lb	59	9.5	417
Non-Dairy Cream				
Rich's Coffee Rich	½ oz	20	2	10
Non-Dairy Frozen Whipped Topping				
Cool Whip	1 tbsp	34	1	0
Cool Whip, Extra Creamy	1 tbsp	16	1	0
Noodles, egg noodles, enriched or unenriched				
dry form	16 oz (1 lb) pkg	1,760	326.6	23
	8 oz pkg	881	163.4	11
cooked	8.8 cups (yield from 1 lb dry)	1,760	326.6	23
	4.4 cups (yield from 8 oz dry)	881	163.4	11
	1 cup	200	37.3	3
	1 lb (yield from approx 5⅛ oz dry)	567	105.7	9
Noodles, chow mein, canned	5 oz can	694	82.4	—
	3 oz can	416	49.3	—
	1 cup	220	26.1	—
Noodles, brand name				
Noodle Roni Parmesano	½ oz dry	130	21	270
Nutmeg, ground	1 tsp	12	1.08	trace
Nuts				
See individual kinds				
Nuts, Mixed, Brand name				
Planters	1 oz	180	6	130
Mixed, Unsalted	1 oz	180	6	0
Dry Roasted, Unsalted	1 oz	170	15	0

Food	Quantity or Portion	Calories	Carbo-hydrates (grams)	Sodium (milli-grams)

O

Oat products used mainly as hot breakfast cereals

Food	Quantity or Portion	Calories	Carbo-hydrates	Sodium
Oat flakes, maple-flavored, instant-cooking (about 1 min cooking time)	1 cup dry form	365	68.7	1
	1 cup cooked	166	31.2	257
oat granules, maple-flavored, regular (about 3 min cooking time)	1 cup dry form	402	76.1	1
	1 cup cooked	147	27.9	176
oat & wheat cereal	1 cup dry form	346	64.9	2
	1 cup cooked	159	29.6	412
oatmeal or rolled oats, regular (5 min or longer cooking time) & instant-cooking (about 1 min cooking time)	1 cup dry form	312	54.6	2
	1 cup cooked	132	23.3	523

Oat products used mainly as ready-to-eat breakfast cereals

Food	Quantity or Portion	Calories	Carbo-hydrates	Sodium
oats, shredded, added protein, sugar, salt, minerals, vitamins	1 cup	171	32.4	275
oats, puffed, added sugar, salt, minerals, vitamins	1 cup	99	18.8	317
oats (with corn), puffed, added salt, minerals, vitamins, sugar-covered	1 cup	139	30.0	206

Ocean Perch, Atlantic (redfish)

Food	Quantity or Portion	Calories	Carbo-hydrates	Sodium
cooked, fried	1 lb	1,030	30.8	694
	1 oz	64	1.9	43
frozen, breaded, fried, reheated (fillet 6¾" long, 1¾" wide, ⅝" thick, wt 3.2 oz)	5 fillets, yield from 1 lb container	1,404	72.6	v
	1 fillet	281	14.5	v
	1 lb	1,447	74.8	v

Oils, salad or cooking

Food	Quantity or Portion	Calories	Carbo-hydrates	Sodium
corn, safflower, soybean oils, sesame, cottonseed oils, soybean-cottonseed oil blend	16 fl oz (1 pt) bottle	3,854	0	0
	24 fl oz (1 pt, 8 oz) bottle	5,781	0	0
	1 qt	7,708	0	0
	1 cup	1,927	0	0
	1 tbsp	120	0	0
olive oil	4 fl oz bottle	955	0	0
	16 fl oz (1 pt) bottle	3,819	0	0
	1 quart	7,638	0	0
	1 cup	1,909	0	0
	1 tbsp	119	0	0
peanut oil	24 fl oz (1 pt 8 oz) bottle	5,728	0	0
	1 qt	7,638	0	0
	1 cup	1,909	0	0
	1 tbsp	119	0	0

Food	Quantity or Portion	Calories	Carbo-hydrates (grams)	Sodium (milli-grams)
Okra				
raw	1 cup, crosscut slices	36	7.6	3
	1 lb	163	34.5	14
cooked (boiled), drained	10 pods, 3″ long, ⅝″ diam	31	6.4	2
	1 cup, crosscut slices	46	9.6	3
	1 lb	132	27.2	9
frozen, cuts & pods, cooked (boiled), drained	9 oz, yield from 10 oz frozen	97	22.4	5
	14.4 oz, yield from 1 lb frozen	155	35.9	8
	1 cup cuts	70	16.3	4
	1 lb	172	39.9	9
Oleomargarine				
See Margarine				
Olives, pickled, canned or bottled				
green				
whole	10 small, 135 per lb	33	.4	686
	10 lg, 98 per lb	45	.5	926
	10 giant, 53–64 per lb	76	.9	1,572
pitted	1 lb pitted	526	5.9	10,886
ripe (black)				
whole	10 small, 135 per lb	38	.8	237
	10 med, 113 per lb	44	.9	280
	10 lg, 98 per lb	51	1.0	322
	10 ex lg, 82 per lb	61	1.2	385
	10 mammoth, 70 per lb	72	1.5	454
	10 giant, 53–60 per lb	89	1.8	559
	10 jumbo, 46–50 per lb	105	2.1	664
	1 cup sliced	174	3.5	1,098
pitted	1 lb, pitted	585	11.8	3,688
ripe, salt cured, oil coated, Greek style				
whole	10 med olives, 188 per lb	65	1.7	631
	10 ex lg, 137 per lb	89	2.3	868
pitted	1 lb, pitted	1,533	39.5	14,914
Olive Oil				
See Oils				
Omelet				
See Eggs, omelet				
Onion Powder	1 tsp	7	1.69	1
Onions, mature (dry)				
raw	1 cup chopped	65	14.8	17
	1 cup grated or ground	89	20.4	24
	1 cup sliced	44	10.0	12

Food	Quantity or Portion	Calories	Carbo-hydrates (grams)	Sodium (milli-grams)
	1 tbsp chopped or minced	4	.9	1
	1 lb	172	39.5	45
cooked (boiled), drained	1 cup whole or sliced	61	13.7	15
	1 lb	132	29.5	32
Onions, young green See Scallions				
Oranges, raw				
California Oranges				
Navels (winter oranges)				
whole fruit	1 lg fruit, 3⁄16″ diam	87	21.8	2
	1 med fruit, 2⅞″ diam	71	17.8	1
	1 small fruit, 2⅜″ diam	45	11.3	1
sections or cup pieces from med fruit	1 cup with membranes	77	19.1	2
	1 cup without membranes	84	21.0	2
	1 cup diced, small pieces	107	26.7	2
Valencias (summer oranges)				
whole fruit	1 lg fruit, 3 1⁄16″ diam	96	23.4	2
	1 med fruit, 2⅝″ diam	62	15.0	1
	1 small fruit, 2⅜″ diam	50	12.2	1
sections or cut pieces from med fruit	1 cup with membranes	79	19.2	2
	1 cup without membranes	92	22.3	2
	1 cup diced, small pieces	107	26.0	2
Florida oranges, average of all commercial varieties				
whole fruit	1 average size fruit, 2⅝″ diam	66	16.9	1
	1 lg fruit, 2 15⁄16″ diam	89	22.6	2
	1 med fruit, 2 11⁄16″ diam	71	18.1	2
	1 small fruit, 2½″ diam	57	14.5	1
sections or cut pieces from med fruit	1 cup without membranes	87	22.2	2
	1 cup with membranes	78	19.8	2
	1 cup diced, small pieces	99	25.2	2
Oranges, raw, used with peel (California Valencias)				
whole fruit, med, 2⅝″ diam	1 orange	64	24.7	3
cut-up fruit, chopped in small pieces	1 cup	68	26.4	3
Orange Juice, fresh, & oranges used for juice				
average of all commercial varieties	1 cup juice	112	25.8	2
	whole fruit used for juice, average, 2⅝″ diam	39	9.0	1

Food	Quantity or Portion	Calories	Carbo-hydrates (grams)	Sodium (milli-grams)
from California oranges				
Navels (winter oranges) (approx 3 to 5 oranges per cup juice, depending on size)	1 cup juice	120	28.1	2
Valencias, (summer oranges) (approx 2–4 oranges per cup juice, depending on size)	1 cup juice	117	26.0	2
from Florida oranges				
average of all commercial varieties	1 cup juice	106	24.7	2
	juice of 1 average fruit, ⅝″ diam, yield approx ⅜ cup juice	41	9.5	1
early & midseason oranges (Hamlin, Parson Brown, Pineapple) (approx 2–3 oranges per cup juice, depending on size)	1 cup juice	98	22.9	2
late season oranges (Valencias) (approx 2–3 oranges per cup juice, depending on size)	1 cup juice	112	26.0	2
Temple oranges (approx 1½–3 oranges per cup juice, depending on size)	1 cup juice	134	32.0	2
Orange Juice, canned				
unsweetened	6 fl oz can	89	20.8	2
	1 cup	120	27.9	2
	1 fl oz	15	3.5	trace
sweetened with nutritive sweetener	6 fl oz can	97	22.8	2
	1 cup	130	30.5	2
	1 fl oz	16	3.8	trace
Orange Juice Concentrate, canned, unsweetened				
undiluted	1 fl oz	84	19.2	2
diluted with 5 parts water by volume	1 cup	114	25.5	2
	1 fl oz	14	3.2	trace
Orange Juice Concentrate, frozen, unsweetened				
undiluted	6 fl oz can, yield 3 cups (24 fl oz) diluted juice	362	86.7	4
diluted with 3 parts water by volume	1 qt	488	115.4	10
	1 cup	122	28.9	2
	6 fl oz glass	92	21.7	2
Orange Juice, dehydrated (crystals)				
dry form	1 oz, yields approx 1 cup juice	108	25.2	2
	1 lb, yields approx 1 gal juice	1,724	403.3	36

Food	Quantity or Portion	Calories	Carbo-hydrates (grams)	Sodium (milli-grams)
prepared with water (1 lb of crystals yields approx 1 gal juice)	1 cup	114	26.8	2
Orange Peel				
raw, grated (med-size grating)	1 tbsp	(a)	1.5	trace
	1 tsp	(a)	.5	trace
	1 oz	(a)	7.1	1
candied	1 oz	90	22.9	—
	1 lb	1,433	365.6	—
Orange-Cranberry Relish				
See Cranberry-orange relish				
Orange Juice & Apricot Juice Drink,	1 cup	125	31.6	trace
canned (approx 40% fruit juices)	6 fl oz glass	94	23.7	trace
	1 fl oz	16	4.0	trace
Oregano	1 tsp	5	0.97	trace
Oysterplant				
See Salsify				
Oysters				
raw (chilled), meat only, drained				
Eastern	12 fl oz can 18–27 Select (med) or 27–44 Standard (small) oysters	224	11.6	248
	1 cup, approx 13–19 Selects (med) or 19–31 Standards (small)	158	8.2	175
	1 lb, approx 19 or less Counts (ex lg); 19–25 Extra Selects (large); 25–36 Selects (medium); 36–59 Standards (small); or over 59 Very Small	299	15.4	331
	1 oz, approx 2 Selects (med) or 3 Standards (small)	19	1.0	21
Pacific	12 oz can, approx 6–9 med or 9–13 small oysters	309	21.8	v
	1 cup, approx 4–6 med or 6–9 small oysters	218	15.4	v
	1 lb (8 or less lg, 8–11 medium, 12–17 small, over 17 extra small)	413	29.0	v
Western (Olympia)	1 lb (275–300 oysters)	413	29.0	v
cooked (fried)	4 Select (med) oysters, approx 3″ long, raw, 1½″ wide long fried	108	8.4	93

(a) Value not calculated because digestibility of raw peel is not known.

Food	Quantity or Portion	Calories	Carbo-hydrates (grams)	Sodium (milli-grams)
	1 oz, approx 2½ Select oysters	68	5.3	58
Oyster Stew, home prepared	1 cup with 1 part oysters to 2 parts milk by volume (approx 6 med oysters per cup)	233	10.8	814
	1 cup with 1 part oysters to 3 parts milk by volume (approx 4 med oysters per cup)	206	11.3	487

P

Food	Quantity or Portion	Calories	Carbo-hydrates (grams)	Sodium (milli-grams)
Pancakes				
Home baked, made with enriched or unenriched flour	1 lg pancake, 6″ diam, ½″ thick (yield from approx 7 tbsp batter)	169	24.9	310
	1 small pancake, 4″ diam, ⅜″ thick (yield from approx 2½ tbsp batter)	62	9.2	115
Made with egg & milk from plain or buttermilk mix, enriched or unenriched flour	1 large pancake, 6″ diam, ½″ thick (yield from approx 7 tbsp batter)	164	23.7	412
	1 small pancake, 4″ diam, ⅜″ thick (yield from approx 2½ tbsp batter)	61	8.7	152
Made with egg & milk from buckwheat and other cereal flour mix	1 lg pancake, 6″ diam, ½″ thick (yield from approx 7 tbsp batter)	146	17.4	339
	1 small pancake, 4″ diam, ⅜″ thick (yield from approx 2½ tbsp batter)	54	6.4	125
Pancake Mix, brand names				
Aunt Jemima				
Buttermilk Pancake and Waffle Mix	¼ cup (equals 3 4″ pancakes)	340	40	990
Buttermilk Complete	½ cup (equals 3 4″ pancakes)	260	51	960
Complete	½ cup (equals 3 4″ pancakes)	280	52	960
Original	¼ cup (equals 3 4″ pancakes)	200	26	550
Whole Wheat	⅓ cup (equals 3 4″ pancakes)	250	32	725
Hungry Jack (Pillsbury)				
Buttermilk Complete	3 4″ pancakes	180	39	710

Food	Quantity or Portion	Calories	Carbo-hydrates (grams)	Sodium (milli-grams)
Extra Light Complete	3 4″ pancakes	180	39	705
Extra Light	3 4″ pancakes	200	26	495
Hungry Jack Pan Shakes	3 4″ pancakes made with water	200	39	840
	3 4″ pancakes made with milk	250	43	880
Papaws, common, North American type, raw	1 whole fruit, 2″ diam, 3¾″ long	83	16.4	—
	1 cup mashed	213	42.0	—
Papayas, raw	1 lb fruit, 3½″ diam, 5⅛″ high, med fruit	119	30.4	9
	1 cup cubed, ½″ pieces	55	14.0	4
	1 lb	177	45.4	14
Paprika	1 tsp	6	0.44	0.08
Parsley, common garden (plain) & curled-leaf varieties, raw	1 cup chopped	26	5.1	27
	1 tbsp, chopped	2	.3	2
	10 sprigs, each approx 2½″ long	4	.9	5
Parsley, dried	1 tsp	1	0.15	1
Parsnips				
raw, prepackaged without tops	1 lb pkg	293	67.5	46
cooked (boiled), drained	1 lg parsnip, 9″ long, 2¼″ diam	106	23.8	13
	1 small parsnip, 6″ long, 1⅛″ diam	23	5.2	3
	1 cup diced or 2″ lengths	102	23.1	12
	1 cup mashed	139	31.3	17
Passion Fruit See Granadilla				
Pasta See Macaroni				
Pastina, egg, enriched, dry form	1 cup	651	122.1	9
Pastry, Danish See Rolls & Breads				
Pastry Shell, plain See Piecrust				
Pate de Foie Gras, canned	1 tbsp	60	.6	v
	1 tsp	18	.2	v
Peaches				
fresh				
whole peeled	1 lg fruit, 2¾″ diam, approx 2½ per lb	58	14.8	2
	1 med fruit, 2½″ diam, approx 4 per lb	38	9.7	1
sliced	1 cup	65	16.5	2
diced	1 cup	70	17.9	2
1 lb	sliced or diced	172	44.0	5

Food	Quantity or Portion	Calories	Carbo-hydrates (grams)	Sodium (milli-grams)
canned, peaches & liquid				
water pack without artificial sweetener, clingstone peaches	8 oz can, halved style	70	18.4	5
	1 lg peach half with 2 tbsp liquid	28	7.4	2
	1 med peach half with 1⅔ tbsp liquid	24	6.2	2
	1 cup, halved or sliced styles	76	19.8	5
syrup pack, heavy	8¾ oz can, halved & sliced styles	193	49.8	5
	16 oz can, halved & sliced styles	354	91.2	9
	1 lg half, 2½ tbsp liquid	85	21.9	2
	1 lg half, 2⅛ tbsp drained liquid	75	19.3	2
	1 small half, 1¾ tbsp drained liquid	63	16.3	2
	1 cup, halved, sliced or chunk styles	200	51.5	5
dehydrated, sulfured, nugget type & pieces				
uncooked	1 cup	340	88.0	21
	1 lb	1,542	399.2	95
cooked, fruit & liquid, with added sugar	1 cup	351	90.8	15
	1 lb	549	142.0	23
dried, sulfured (halves)				
uncooked	11–12 oz container	854	222.7	52
	1 cup	419	109.3	26
	10 lg halves	380	99.0	23
	10 med halves	341	88.8	21
cooked, fruit & liquid				
without added sugar	1 cup	205	53.5	13
	1 lb	372	97.1	23
with added sugar	1 cup	321	83.2	11
	1 lb	540	139.7	18
frozen, sliced, sweetened with nutritive sweetener, not thawed	10 oz container	250	64.2	6
	1 cup	220	56.5	5
	1 lb	399	102.5	9
Peach Nectar, canned (approx 40% fruit)	5½ fl oz can	82	21.2	2
	12 fl oz can	179	46.3	4
	1 cup	120	30.9	2
	6 fl oz glass	90	23.2	2
	1 fl oz	15	3.9	trace
Peanuts				
roasted in shell (with skins)				
whole	1 lb (yields approx 10.7 oz shelled nuts)	1,769	62.6	15
	10 jumbo nuts	105	3.7	1
shelled, chopped	1 cup	838	29.7	7
	1 tbsp	52	1.9	trace

Food	Quantity or Portion	Calories	Carbo-hydrates (grams)	Sodium (milli-grams)
roasted, salted	1 cup whole, halves or chopped	842	27.1	602
	1 lb	2,654	85.3	1,896
	1 oz	166	5.3	119
Peanuts, brand name				
Planters				
Cocktail	1 oz	170	5	160
Cocktail, Unsalted	1 oz	170	5	0
Dry Roasted	1 oz	160	6	250
Honey Roasted	1 oz	170	8	180
Peanut Butter, brand names				
Jif Creamy	2 tbsp	190	6	155
Jif Extra Chunky	2 tbsp	190	6	130
Peter Pan Creamy	2 tbsp	180	5	150
Peter Pan Crunchy	2 tbsp	180	5	150
Skippy Creamy	2 tbsp	190	4	150
Skippy Super Chunky	2 tbsp	190	4	130
Peanut Flour, defatted	1 cup	223	18.9	5
Peanut Oil				
See Oils				
Pears				
raw, including skin				
whole				
Bartlett, 2½″ diam, 3½″ high (approx 2½ per lb)	1 pear	100	25.1	3
Bosc,	2½″ diam, 3½″ high (approx 3 per lb)	86	21.6	3
sliced or cubed	1 cup	101	25.2	3
	1 lb	277	69.4	9
canned, pears & liquid				
water pack, without artificial sweetener	8 oz can (approx contents 5 pears & 5 tbsp liquid)	73	18.8	2
	1 pear half with 1 tbsp liquid	14	3.7	trace
	1 cup	78	20.3	2
syrup pack, heavy	8½ oz can (approx contents 5 pears & 5 tbsp liquid)	183	47.2	2
	1 pear half with 1 tbsp liquid	36	9.4	trace
	1 cup	194	50.0	3
dried, sulfured (halves)				
uncooked	1 cup	482	121.1	13
	1 lb, approx 26 halves	1,216	305.3	32
	10 halves	469	117.8	12
cooked fruit & liquid				
without added sugar	1 cup	321	80.8	8
	1 lb	572	143.8	14
with added sugar	1 cup	423	106.4	8
	1 lb	685	172.4	14

PEAS

Food	Quantity or Portion	Calories	Carbo-hydrates (grams)	Sodium (milli-grams)
Pear Nectar, canned (approx 40% fruit)	5½ fl oz can	89	22.7	2
	12 fl oz can	195	49.5	4
	1 cup	130	33.0	3
	6 fl oz glass	97	24.7	2
	1 fl oz	16	4.1	trace
Peas, green, fresh				
raw	1 cup	122	20.9	3
	1 lb (yields approx 2⅔ cups cooked peas)	381	65.3	9
cooked (boiled), drained	1 cup	114	19.4	2
	1 lb, yield from approx 2¾ lb peas in pod or 1¹⁄₁₆ lb shelled peas	322	54.9	5
Peas, green, canned				
Early or June peas				
regular pack, peas & liquid	8½ oz can	159	30.1	569
	1 can or jar	318	60.3	1,138
	1 cup	164	31.1	588
	1 lb	299	56.7	1,070
regular pack, drained peas	5½ oz peas, yield from 8½ oz can	138	26.4	371
	11 oz peas, yield from 17 oz can	275	52.6	739
	1 cup	150	28.6	401
	1 lb	399	76.2	1,070
special dietary pack (low sodium), peas & liquid	8½ oz can	133	23.6	7
	17 oz can or jar	265	47.2	14
	1 cup	137	24.4	7
	1 lb	249	44.5	14
special dietary pack (low sodium), drained peas	5½ oz peas, yield from 8½ oz can	122	22.5	5
	11 oz peas, yield from 17 oz can	244	44.8	9
	1 cup	133	24.3	5
	1 lb	354	64.9	14
Sweet peas				
regular pack, peas & liquid	8½ oz can	137	25.1	569
	17 oz can or jar	275	50.1	1,138
	1 cup	142	25.9	588
	1 lb	259	47.2	1,070
regular pack, drained peas	5½ oz peas, yield from 8½ oz can	126	23.6	371
	11 oz peas, yield from 17 oz can	250	47.0	739
	1 cup	136	25.5	401
	1 lb	363	68.0	1,070
special dietary pack (low sodium), peas & liquid	8½ oz can	113	19.8	7
	17 oz can or jar	227	39.5	14
	1 cup	117	20.4	7
	1 lb	213	37.2	14

Food	Quantity or Portion	Calories	Carbo-hydrates (grams)	Sodium (milli-grams)
special dietary pack (low sodium), drained peas	5½ oz peas, yield from 8½ oz can	113	20.4	5
	11 oz peas, yield from 17 oz can	225	40.7	9
	1 cup	122	22.1	5
	1 lb	327	59.0	14
Peas, green, frozen				
cooked (boiled), drained	2½ cups, yield from 1 lb frozen	275	47.7	465
	1.6 cups, yield from 10 oz frozen	172	29.9	291
	1 cup	109	18.9	184
	1 lb, yield from approx 1 lb, 2 oz frozen	308	53.5	522
Peas, mature seeds, dry				
whole				
raw	1 cup	680	120.6	70
	1 lb	1,542	273.5	159
split, without seedcoat				
raw	1 cup	696	125.4	80
	1 lb	1,579	284.4	181
cooked	1 cup	230	41.6	26
	1 lb	522	94.3	59
Peas & Carrots, frozen				
cooked (boiled), drained	2¾ cups, yield from 1 lb frozen	236	44.9	374
	1¾ cups, yield from 10 oz frozen	147	28.1	234
	1 cup	85	16.2	134
	1 lb, yield from 1⅓ lb frozen	240	45.8	381
Pecans				
in shell	10 oversize nuts, 55 or less per lb	299	6.4	trace
	10 ex lg nuts, 56–63 per lb	277	5.9	trace
	10 lg nuts, 64–77 per lb	236	5.0	trace
	1 lb, yields approx 8.5 oz shelled nuts	1,652	35.1	trace
shelled	1 cup, halves	742	15.8	trace
	1 cup, chopped	811	17.2	trace
	1 tbsp, chopped	52	1.1	trace
	1 cup, ground	653	13.9	trace
	1 lb (yield from approx 1.9 lb in shell)	3,116	66.2	trace
	1 oz	195	4.1	trace
Pepper, Black	1 tsp	5	1.36	1
Pepper, Red or Cayenne	1 tsp	6	1.02	1
Pepper, White	1 tsp	7	1.65	.03

Food	Quantity or Portion	Calories	Carbo-hydrates (grams)	Sodium (milli-grams)
Peppers, hot, chili				
immature, green				
canned, chili sauce	1 cup	49	12.3	—
mature, red				
canned, chili sauce	1 cup	51	9.6	—
dried, chili powder with added seasoning	1 tsp	7	1.1	31
Peppers, sweet, garden varieties				
immature, green				
raw				
whole	1 fancy grade, 3¾" long, 3" diam, approx 2¼ per lb	36	7.9	21
	1 no. 1 grade, 2¾" long, 2½" diam, 5 per lb	16	3.5	10
cut into strips	1 cup	22	4.8	13
chopped or diced	1 cup	33	7.2	20
ring	1 ring, 3" diam, ¼" thick,	2	.5	1
	1 lb, sliced, chopped or diced or cut into strips	100	21.8	59
cooked				
boiled, drained	1 Fancy grade pepper	29	6.1	14
	1 no. 1 grade pepper	13	2.8	7
	1 cup strips	24	5.1	12
	1 lb	82	17.2	41
stuffed with beef & crumbs (pepper, 2¾" long, 2½" diam with 1⅛ cups stuffing)	1 stuffed pepper	315	31.1	581
Peppers, sweet, red (mature)				
whole	1 Fancy grade pepper, 3¾" long, 3" diam, approx 2¼ per lb	51	11.6	—
	1 no. 1 grade pepper, 2¾" long, 2½" diam, approx 5 per lb	23	5.2	—
cut into strips	1 cup	31	7.1	—
chopped or diced	1 cup	47	10.7	—
ring	3" diam, ¼" thick ring	3	.7	—
	1 lb	141	32.2	—
Perch				
See Ocean Perch				
Persimmons, raw				
Japanese, or kaki, 2½" diam, 3" high	1 fruit	129	33.1	10
native	1 fruit	31	8.2	trace

Food	Quantity or Portion	Calories	Carbo-hydrates (grams)	Sodium (milli-grams)
Pickles, cucumber				
dill or sour				
whole	1 lg, approx 4″ long, 1¾″ diam	15	3.0	1,928
	1 med, approx 3¾″ long, 1¼″ diam	7	1.4	928
spears or sticks, each piece approx 6″ long	1 spear	3	.7	428
sliced crosswise, each piece 1½″ diam, ¼″ thick	1 cup (approx 23 slices)	17	3.4	2,213
	2 slices	1	.3	186
Fresh, sweetened with nutritive sweetener (bread-and-butter pickles); slices, 1½″ diam, ¼″ thick	1 cup, approx 23 slices	124	30.4	1,144
	2 slices	11	2.7	101
Sweet (sweetened with nutritive sweetener)				
whole, gherkins	1 lg (approx 3″ long)	51	12.8	—
	1 small (approx 2½″ long)	22	5.5	—
	1 midget, approx 2⅛″ long)	9	2.2	—
chopped, approx ¼″ cubes	1 cup	234	58.4	—
Chowchow or mustard pickles (cucumber with added cauliflower, onion, mustard)	1 cup, sour	70	9.8	3,211
	1 cup, sweet	284	66.2	1,291
Relish, finely cut or chopped, sweet	1 cup	338	83.3	1,744
	1 tbsp	21	5.1	107
	1 restaurant packet, approx ⅔ tbsp	14	3.4	71
Pies (Baked, piecrust made with unenriched flour (9″ diam))				
Apple				
pie, whole	1 pie	2,419	360.0	2,844
lg slice 4¾″ arc	(⅙ pie)	404	60.2	476
med slice 3½″ arc	(⅛ pie)	302	45.0	355
sector, 1″ arc		86	12.7	101
Banana Custard				
pie, whole	1 pie	2,011	279.4	1,765
lg slice 4¾″ arc	(⅙ pie)	336	46.7	295
med slice 3½″ arc	(⅛ pie)	252	35.0	221
sector, 1″ arc		71	9.9	62
Blackberry				
pie, whole	1 pie	2,296	325.1	2,533
lg slice 4¾″ arc	(⅙ pie)	384	54.4	423
med slice 3½″ arc	(⅛ pie)	287	40.6	316
sector, 1″ arc		81	11.5	90
Blueberry				
pie, whole	1 pie	2,287	329.8	2,533
lg slice 4¾″ arc	(⅙ pie)	382	55.1	423
med slice 3½″ arc	(⅛ pie)	286	41.2	316
sector, 1″ arc		81	11.7	90

Food	Quantity or Portion	Calories	Carbo-hydrates (grams)	Sodium (milli-grams)
Boston Cream				
See Cakes				
Butterscotch				
pie, whole	1 pie	2,430	348.5	1,947
lg slice 4¾" arc	(⅙ pie)	406	58.2	325
med slice 3½" arc	(⅛ pie)	304	43.7	244
sector, 1" arc		86	12.3	69
Cherry				
pie, whole	1 pie	2,466	362.9	2,873
lg slice 4¾" arc	(⅙ pie)	412	60.7	480
med slice 3½" arc	(⅛ pie)	308	45.3	350
sector, 1" arc		87	12.8	102
Chocolate Chiffon				
pie, whole	1 pie	2,125	283.2	1,633
lg slice 4¾" arc	(⅙ pie)	354	47.2	272
med slice 3½" arc	(⅛ pie)	266	35.4	204
sector, 1" arc		75	10.0	58
Chocolate Meringue				
pie, whole	1 pie	2,293	304.9	2,330
lg slice 4¾" arc	(⅙ pie)	383	50.9	389
med slice 3½" arc	(⅛ pie)	287	38.2	292
sector, 1" arc		81	10.8	82
Coconut Custard				
pie, whole	1 pie	2,139	226.6	2,248
lg slice 4¾" arc	(⅙ pie)	357	37.8	375
med slice 3½" arc	(⅛ pie)	268	28.4	282
sector, 1" arc		76	8.0	80
Custard				
pie, whole	1 pie	1,984	212.0	2,612
lg slice 4¾" arc	(⅙ pie)	331	35.6	436
med slice 3½" arc	(⅛ pie)	249	26.7	327
sector, 1" arc		70	7.5	92
Lemon Chiffon				
pie, whole	1 pie	2,028	283.8	1,691
lg slice 4¾" arc	(⅙ pie)	338	47.3	282
med slice 3½" arc	(⅛ pie)	254	35.5	211
sector, 1" arc		72	10.0	60
Lemon Meringue				
pie, whole	1 pie	2,142	316.7	2,369
lg slice 4¾" arc	(⅙ pie)	357	52.8	395
med slice 3½" arc	(⅛ pie)	268	39.6	296
sector, 1" arc		76	11.2	84
Mince				
pie, whole	1 pie	2,561	389.3	4,234
lg slice 4¾" arc	(⅙ pie)	428	65.1	708
med slice 3½" arc	(⅛ pie)	320	48.6	529
sector, 1" arc		91	13.8	150
Peach				
pie, whole	1 pie	2,410	361.0	2,533
lg slice 4¾" arc	(⅙ pie)	403	60.4	423
med slice 3½" arc	(⅛ pie)	301	45.1	316
sector, 1" arc		85	12.8	90

Food	Quantity or Portion	Calories	Carbo-hydrates (grams)	Sodium (milli-grams)
Pecan				
pie, whole	1 pie	3,449	423.2	1,823
lg slice 4¾" arc	(⅙ pie)	577	70.8	305
med slice 3½" arc	(⅛ pie)	431	52.8	228
sector, 1" arc		122	15.0	65
Pineapple				
pie, whole	1 pie	2,391	360.0	2,561
lg slice 4¾" arc	(⅙ pie)	400	60.2	428
med slice 3½" arc	(⅛ pie)	299	45.0	320
sector, 1" arc		85	12.7	91
Pineapple Chiffon				
pie, whole	1 pie	1,866	253.4	1,659
lg slice 4¾" arc	(⅙ pie)	311	42.2	276
med slice 3½" arc	(⅛ pie)	233	31.7	207
sector, 1" arc		66	9.0	59
Pineapple Custard				
pie, whole	1 pie	2,002	292.1	1,693
lg slice 4¾" arc	(⅙ pie)	334	48.8	283
med slice 3½" arc	(⅛ pie)	251	36.6	212
sector, 1" arc		71	10.3	60
Pumpkin				
pie, whole	1 pie	1,920	223.0	1,947
lg slice 4¾" arc	(⅙ pie)	321	37.2	325
med slice 3½" arc	(⅛ pie)	241	27.9	244
sector, 1" arc		68	7.9	69
Raisin				
pie, whole	1 pie	2,552	406.4	2,693
lg slice 4¾" arc	(⅙ pie)	427	67.9	450
med slice 3½" arc	(⅛ of pie)	319	50.7	336
sector, 1" arc		90	14.4	95
Rhubarb				
pie, whole	1 pie	2,391	361.0	2,552
lg slice 4¾" arc	(⅙ pie)	400	60.4	427
med slice 3½" arc	(⅛ pie)	299	45.1	319
sector, 1" arc		85	12.8	90
Strawberry				
pie, whole	1 pie	1,469	229.3	1,439
lg slice 4¾" arc	(⅙ pie)	246	38.3	241
med slice 3½" arc	(⅛ pie)	184	28.7	180
sector, 1" arc		52	8.1	51
Sweet potato				
pie, whole	1 pie	1,938	215.7	1,984
lg slice 4 ¾" arc	(⅙ pie)	324	36.0	331
med slice 3½" arc	(⅛ pie)	243	27.0	249
sector, 1" arc		60	7.6	70
Pies, Frozen in unbaked form (8" diam, net wt 20 oz, (1 lb 4 oz) to 26 oz (1 lb 10 oz)				
Apple				
unbaked or baked pie	1 pie	1,386	219.1	1,168
lg slice 4⅛" arc	(⅙ pie)	231	36.5	195

Food	Quantity or Portion	Calories	Carbo-hydrates (grams)	Sodium (milli-grams)
med slice 3⅛″ arc	(⅛ pie)	173	27.4	146
sector, 1″ arc		55	8.7	47
Cherry				
unbaked or baked pie	1 pie	1,690	257.4	1,333
lg slice 4⅛″ arc	(⅙ pie)	282	42.9	222
med slice 3⅛″ arc	(⅛ pie)	211	32.2	167
sector, 1″ arc		67	10.3	53
Coconut Custard, baked	1 pie	1,494	177.0	1,512
lg slice 4⅛″ arc	(⅙ pie)	249	29.5	252
med slice 3⅛″ arc	(⅛ pie)	187	22.1	189
sector, 1″ arc		60	7.1	60
Pies, Frozen, brand names				
Weight Watchers				
Apple Pie	3 oz	180	33.0	290
Cherry Pie	3 oz	180	33.0	290
Pies, Prepared from mix (filling & piecrust), baked				
Coconut Custard Pie (filling made with mix, egg yolks, milk), 8″ diam	1 whole pie	1,618	231.9	1,873
lg slice 4⅛″ arc	(⅙ of pie)	270	38.7	313
med slice 3⅛″ arc	(⅛ of pie)	203	29.1	235
sector, 1″ arc		65	9.3	75
Piecrust or plain pastry, made with enriched or unenriched flour				
unbaked	1 pie shell	900	79.0	1,102
baked	1 pie shell	900	78.8	1,100
Piecrust mix	1 10 oz pkg	1,482	140.6	1,968
Piecrust, prepared with water, baked from mix (yield from 10 oz pkg)	1 piecrust, 11.3 oz	1,485	140.8	2,602
Piecrust Mix, brand names				
Betty Crocker Pie Crust Mix	⅟₁₆ pkg (equals ⅛ pie)	120	10	140
Bisquick Buttermilk Baking Mix	2 oz (approx ½ cup)	240	37	700
Pigs' feet, pickled	2 oz	113	0	—
Pimentos, canned, solids & liquid	4 oz can or jar	31	6.6	—
	2 oz jar	15	3.3	—
	1 lb	122	26.3	—
Pineapple				
raw	1 cup, diced pieces	81	21.2	2
	1 slice, 3½″ diam ¾″ thick	44	11.5	1
	1 lb (approx 3 cups diced pieces or 5½ slices)	236	62.1	5
candied				
prepackaged slices & chunks	4 oz container, 2 slices or approx ½ cup chunks	357	90.4	—
	8 oz container (4			

Food	Quantity or Portion	Calories	Carbo-hydrates (grams)	Sodium (milli-grams)
	slices or 1 cup chunks)	717	181.6	—
	1 oz	90	22.7	—
canned, pineapple & liquid				
water pack, without artificial	1 cup	96	25.1	2
sweetener	1 lb	177	46.3	5
syrup pack				
heavy	8¼ oz can	173	45.4	2
	1 cup, chunk tidbits, crushed styles	189	49.5	3
	1 med slice, 3" diam, 5/16" thick	43	11.3	1
	1 lb	336	88.0	5
extra heavy	8¾ oz can	223	58.0	2
	1 cup, chunk or crushed styles	234	60.8	3
	1 med slice, 3" diam, 5/16" thick	52	13.6	1
	1 lb	408	106.1	5
Frozen chunks, sweetened with	13½ oz can	326	85.0	8
nutritive sweetener, not	1 cup	208	54.4	5
thawed	1 lb	386	100.7	9
Pineapple Juice				
canned, unsweetened	6 fl oz can	103	25.4	2
	1 cup	138	33.8	3
	1 fl oz	17	4.2	trace
frozen concentrate, unsweetened	6 fl oz can (yields 3 cups diluted juice)	387	95.7	6
diluted with 3 parts water by	1 cup	130	32.0	3
volume	6 fl oz glass	97	23.9	2
	1 fl oz	16	4.0	trace
Pineapple Juice & grapefruit juice	6 fl oz can	101	25.4	trace
drink, canned (approx 50% fruit	1 cup	135	34.0	trace
juice)	1 fl oz	17	4.3	trace
Pineapple Juice & orange juice	6 fl oz glass	101	25.2	trace
drink, canned (approx 40% fruit	1 cup	135	33.8	trace
juice)	1 fl oz	17	4.2	trace
Pinenuts				
pignolias, shelled	1 oz	156	3.3	—
pinon	1 lb in shell	1,671	53.9	—
	1 oz shelled	180	5.8	—
Pistachio Nuts	1 lb in shell	1,347	43.1	—
	1 lb shelled	2,694	86.2	—
Pizza				
from home recipe, baked (in 14" diam pan)				
with cheese topping	1 whole pizza	1,227	147.2	3,650
	1 sector, 5⅓" arc, ⅛ pizza	153	18.4	456
	1 sector, 1" arc	28	3.4	84
with sausage topping	1 whole pizza	1,252	158.4	3,900

Food	Quantity or Portion	Calories	Carbo-hydrates (grams)	Sodium (milli-grams)
	1 sector, 5⅓″ arc, ⅛ pizza	157	19.8	488
	1 sector, 1″ arc	29	3.7	90
frozen, with cheese				
partially baked or baked	15 oz, 10″ diam pizza	973	140.7	2,571
	5¼″ diam pizza	179	25.8	472
	1 lb	1,039	150.1	2,744
Plantain (baking banana), **raw**	1 fruit, 11″ long, 1⅞″ diam	313	82.0	13
	1 lb	540	141.5	23
Plums, raw				
Damson				
whole	1 cup	87	23.5	3
	10 1″ diam fruits	66	17.8	2
	1 lb	272	73.5	8
pitted	1 cup, halves	112	30.3	3
	1 lb	299	80.7	9
Japanese and hybrid				
whole	1 fruit, 2⅛″ diam	32	8.1	1
	1 lb	205	52.4	4
pitted	1 cup, halves	89	22.8	2
	1 lb	218	55.8	5
Prune type				
whole	1 fruit, 1½″ diam	21	5.6	trace
	1 lb	320	84.0	4
pitted	1 cup, halves	124	32.5	2
	1 lb	340	89.4	5
Plums, canned, fruit & liquid, purple (Italian prunes), whole, unpitted				
water pack, without artificial	1 lb can	198	51.3	9
sweetener	1 cup	114	29.6	5
	3 plums with 2 tbsp liquid	44	11.3	2
syrup pack, heavy	17 oz can	377	98.1	5
	1 cup	214	57.8	3
	1 lb	358	93.1	4
	3 plums with 2¾ tbsp liquid	110	28.7	1
Poha				
See Ground-cherries				
Pokeberry (poke) shoots, unsalted, cooked (boiled), drained	1 cup	33	5.1	—
Pollock, cooked, creamed	1 cup	320	10.0	278
	1 lb	581	18.1	503
Pomegranate, raw, 3⅜″ diam, 2¾″ high	1 fruit	97	25.3	5
Ponderosa Steakhouse				
Imperial Prime Rib	14 oz	572	0	141.2
King Prime Rib	10 oz	409	0	100.6
Prime Rib	7 oz	286	0	70.6
T-Bone	10 oz	240	0	545

Food	Quantity or Portion	Calories	Carbo-hydrates (grams)	Sodium (milli-grams)
New York Strip	8 oz	362	0	79.2
Super Sirloin	10 oz	383	0	695.2
Sirloin	5⅓ oz	197	0	372
Sirloin Tips	5 oz	192.4	0	374.6
Filet Mignon	5 oz	152	0.15	82
Ribeye	4¼ oz	197	0	271
Shrimp	7 pieces	220	9.8	182
Baked fish	4.9 oz	268	11.6	363
Big Chopped Beef	6.8 oz patty	295	0	81
Double Deluxe	2 4 oz patties	362	0	99.1
Child's Square Shooter	1 junior patty	98	0	26.9
Hot Dog With Bun	1 hot dog	248	20.9	805
Baked Potato	7.2 oz	145	32.8	6
French Fries	3 oz	230.4	30.2	4.8
Poppy Seed	1 tsp	15	.66	1
Pop-Tarts (Kellogg's)				
All flavors	1 tart	200(a)	38(a)	220(a)
Popcorn				
unpopped	1 cup	742	147.8	6
popped (commercial)	1 cup lg kernel, plain	23	4.6	trace
	1 cup lg kernel, oil & salt added	41	5.3	175
	1 cup sugar coated	134	29.9	trace
Popcorn, Microwave, brand names				
Orville Redenbacher's Microwave Popping Corn				
Butter Flavor, salt-free	4 cups (10 cups per bag)	140	16	0
Natural flavor	4 cups	140	16	310
Pop-Secret	4 cups	200	21	350
TV Time Microwave Gourmet Popping Corn	4 cups	310	23	250
Popovers, baked (home recipe with enriched flour), 2¾" diam at top, 2" diam at bottom, 4" ht at center (yield from approx ¼ cup batter)	1 popover	90	10.3	88
Pork, fresh, retail cuts				
Ham, fresh				
See Ham				
Loin chops, broiled				
cooked, lean with fat	8.2 oz (yield from 1 lb raw chops with bone)	911	0	141
	10.4 oz (yield from 1 lb raw chops without bone)	1,153	0	179
	2.7 oz chop, cut 3 per lb	305	0	47
	2 oz chop, cut 4 per lb	227	0	35

(a) Content may vary slightly depending on flavor.

Food	Quantity or Portion	Calories	Carbo-hydrates (grams)	Sodium (milli-grams)
lean, trimmed of separable fat	5.9 oz (yield from 1 lb raw chops with bone)	454	0	126
	7.5 oz (yield from 1 lb raw chops without bone)	572	0	159
	2 oz chop, cut 3 per lb	151	0	42
	1½ oz chop, cut 4 per lb	113	0	32
Loin roast, baked or roasted cooked, lean with fat	8.6 oz (yield from 1 lb raw loin with bone)	883	0	147
	10.9 oz (yield from 1 lb raw loin without bone)	1,115	0	185
	1 cup, chopped or diced pieces (not packed)	507	0	84
	1 lb	1,642	0	272
	1 piece, ¼ lb	410	0	68
lean, trimmed of separable fat	6.9 oz (yield from 1 lb raw loin with bone)	495	0	140
	8.7 oz (yield from 1 lb raw loin without bone)	627	0	178
	1 cup chopped or diced pieces (not packed)	356	0	101
	1 lb	1,152	0	327
	1 piece ¼ lb	288	0	82
Shoulder cuts (Boston butt & picnic)				
Boston butt, cooked (roasted) Lean with fat	10.2 oz (yield from 1 lb raw meat with bone & skin)	1,204	0	160
	10.9 oz (yield from 1 lb raw meat without bone & skin)	1,087	0	170
	1 piece, ¼ lb	400	0	63
lean, trimmed of separable fat	8.1 oz (yield from 1 lb raw meat with bone & skin)	559	0	151
	8.6 oz (yield from 1 lb raw meat without bone & skin)	595	0	161
	1 lb	1,107	0	300
	1 piece, ¼ lb	277	0	75
Picnic, cooked (simmered), lean with fat	8.4 oz (yield from 1 lb raw with bone & skin)	890	0	97

Food	Quantity or Portion	Calories	Carbo-hydrates (grams)	Sodium (milli-grams)
	10.2 oz (yield from 1 lb without bone & skin)	1,085	0	118
	1 lb	1,696	0	184
	1 piece, ¼ lb	424	0	46
lean, trimmed of separable fat	6.2 oz (yield from 1 lb raw with bone & skin)	373	0	89
	7.6 oz (yield from 1 lb raw without bone & skin)	456	0	109
	1 lb	962	0	230
	1 piece, ¼ lb	240	0	58
Spareribs, cooked (braised), lean meat with fat	6.3 oz (yield from 1 lb raw)	792	0	65
	1 lb	1,996	0	165
	¼ lb	500	0	41
Pork, cured				
See Bacon, also Ham				
Pork and Beans, canned, brand names				
See also Beans, baked, brand names				
Campbell Pork and Beans	8 oz	250	44	980
Heinz Pork and Beans in Tomato Sauce	8 oz	230	43	1,060
Van Camp Pork and Beans	8 oz	220	41	1,000
Pork sausage				
See Sausage, cold cuts, & luncheon meats				
Potatoes				
See also Potato Mixes, brand names				
Potatoes, cooked				
baked in skin	1 potato, long type, 2⅓″ diam, 4¾″ long (dimensions uncooked)	145	32.8	6
	1 lb	325	73.7	14
boiled in skin, whole	1 long type potato with skin, 2⅓″ diam, 4¾″ long	173	38.9	7
	1 round type potato with skin, 2½″ diam (med size, approx 3 per lb)	104	23.3	4
	1 lb	314	70.6	12
	1 cup diced or sliced	118	26.5	5
	1 lb	345	77.6	14
boiled, hard peeled before cooking (dimensions apply to uncooked potato)	1 long type potato, 2⅓″ diam, 4¾″ long	146	32.6	5
	1 round type potato, 2½″ diam	88	19.6	3

Food	Quantity or Portion	Calories	Carbo-hydrates (grams)	Sodium (milli-grams)
	1 cup diced or sliced	101	22.5	3
	1 lb	295	65.8	9
French fried				
strips 3½" to 4"	10 strips	214	28.1	5
strips 2½" to 3"	10 strips	137	18.0	3
	1 lb	1,243	163.3	27
fried from raw (pan fried)	1 cup	456	55.4	379
	1 lb	1,216	147.9	1,012
hashed brown	1 cup	355	45.1	446
	1 lb	1,039	132.0	1,306
mashed, milk added	1 cup	137	27.3	632
	1 lb	295	59.0	1,365
mashed, milk & table fat added	1 cup	197	25.8	695
	1 lb	426	55.8	1,501
scalloped & au gratin				
with cheese	1 cup	355	33.3	1,095
	1 lb	658	61.7	2,028
without cheese	1 cup	255	36.0	870
	1 lb	472	66.7	1,610
Potatoes, dehydrated mashed (prepared mix)				
flakes without milk—prepared with water, milk, table fat, salt added	1 cup	195	30.5	485
	1 lb	422	65.8	1,048
granules without milk—prepared with water, milk, table fat, salt added	1 cup	202	30.2	538
	1 lb	435	65.3	1,161
granules with milk—prepared with water, milk, table fat, salt added	1 cup	166	27.5	491
	1 lb	358	59.4	1,061
Potatoes, frozen				
hashed brown, cooked	1⅓ cups, yield from 12 oz frozen hashed brown	459	59.5	613
	1 cup	347	45.0	463
	1 lb	1,016	131.5	1,356
French fried, ovenheated (straight-cut and crinkle-cut strips, with cross section approx ½ × ½")	7 oz (yield from 9 oz frozen)	434	66.6	8
	12⅔ oz (yield from 1 lb frozen)	771	118.4	14
	24⅘ oz, yield from 2 lb frozen	1,542	236.7	27
	10 lg strips (3½" to 4")	172	26.3	3
	10 med strips (2" to 3½")	110	16.9	2
	10 small strips (1"–2")	77	11.8	1
	1 lb	998	152.9	18
Potato Chips (smooth or crinkly)	10 chips	114	10.0	—
	1 lb	2,576	226.8	—
	1 oz	161	14.2	—

Food	Quantity or Portion	Calories	Carbo-hydrates (grams)	Sodium (milli-grams)
Potato Chips, name brands				
Herr's				
Dip Style	1 oz	140	16	180
Fresh Crisp	1 oz	140	16	180
Lay's				
Bar-B-Q	1 oz	150	15	360
Potato Chips	1 oz	150	14	200
Sour Cream & Onion	1 oz	150	15	320
Pringle's Potato Chips	1 oz	170	12	250
Ruffles				
Bar-B-Q	1 oz	150	15	290
Potato Chips	1 oz	150	15	200
Sour Cream & Onion	1 oz	150	15	260
Wise Natural Flavor	1 oz	160	14	190
Potato Mixes, brand names				
Betty Crocker				
Au Gratin	⅙ pkg, prepared according to instructions	150	21	630
Buds	⅓ cup for ½ cup serving	130	50	355
Chicken & Herb	⅙ pkg, prepared according to instructions	120	19	585
Hashed Brown with Onions	⅙ pkg prepared according to instructions	160	24	460
Scalloped	⅙ pkg prepared according to instructions	140	19	570
Sour Cream & Chive	⅙ pkg prepared according to instructions	160	21	530
French's				
Cheese Scalloped	½ cup prepared according to instructions	140	20	370
Creamy Italian with Parmesan Sauce	½ cup prepared according to instructions	120	20	540
Idaho Mashed	½ cup prepared according to instructions	120	16	330
Potato Pancakes	3 oz serving (3 3″ pancakes)	130	17	490
Hungry Jack	½ cup (4 oz) prepared according to instructions	40	17	380
Potato Salad, homemade, made with cooked salad dressing, seasonings	1 cup	248	40.8	1,320
	1 lb	449	73.9	2,395
made with mayonnaise & french dressing, hard-boiled eggs, seasonings	1 cup	363	33.5	1,200
	1 lb	658	60.8	2,177
Potato Sticks, ¾–2¾″ long with cross section ⅛ × ⅛″	1 cup	190	17.8	—
	1 lb	2,468	230.4	—
	1 oz	154	14.4	—

Food	Quantity or Portion	Calories	Carbo-hydrates (grams)	Sodium (milli-grams)
Pretzels				
See also Pretzels, brand name	11 oz pkg, rings or logs	1,217	236.8	5,242
	10 oz pkg, rings, thins, rods or sticks	1,108	215.6	4,771
	8 oz pkg, sticks	885	172.3	3,814
	1 oz pkt, approx 45 sticks	111	21.5	476
twisted pretzels	1 Dutch pretzel, 2¾ × 2⅝ × ⅝"	62	12.1	269
	10 1 ring pretzels, 1½" diam	78	15.2	336
	10 3 ring pretzels, each 1⅞ × 1¾ × ¼"	117	22.8	504
straight type pretzels	10 pretzel logs, each 3" long, ½" diam	195	38.0	840
	1 pretzel rod, 7½–7¾" long, ½" diam	55	10.6	235
	10 pretzel sticks 2¼" long, approx ⅛" diam	12	2.3	50
	1 lb	1,769	344.3	7,620
Pretzels, brand names				
Bachman				
Petites	1 oz	110	21	410
Rods	1 oz	110	21	240
Stix	1 oz	93	19	610
Twist	1 oz	110	21	410
Herr's Extra Thin	1 oz	100	22	450
Mr. Salty Twists	1 oz	110	21	585
Reisman				
Rings, unsalted	1 oz	110	23	63
Thin	1 oz	110	23	363
Rold gold				
Rods	1 oz	110	22	510
Sticks	1 oz	110	22	680
Tiny Tim	1 oz	110	22	570
Twists	1 oz	110	23	500
Prunes				
dehydrated, nugget type & pieces				
uncooked	1 cup	344	91.3	11
	1 lb	1,560	414.1	50
cooked, fruit & liquid with	1 cup	504	131.9	11
added sugar	1 lb	816	213.6	18
dried, uncooked				
whole, with pits				
ex lg size (not more than 43	1 lb	1,018	269.1	32
per lb)	10 prunes	274	72.4	9
lg size (not more than 53	1 lb	1,006	266.0	32
per lb)	10 prunes	215	56.9	7

Food	Quantity or Portion	Calories	Carbo-hydrates (grams)	Sodium (milli-grams)
med size (not more than 67 per lb)	1 lb	995	262.9	31
	10 prunes	164	43.5	5
all sizes	1 cup	411	108.5	13
whole, without pits	12 oz container	867	229.2	27
	1 cup	459	121.3	14
	10 prunes	260	68.7	8
	1 lb	1,157	305.7	36
chopped or ground	1 cup, not packed	408	107.8	13
	1 cup, packed	663	175.2	21
dried, cooked, fruit & liquid				
without added sugar	1 cup	253	66.7	9
	1 lb	459	121.1	15
with added sugar	1 cup	409	107.3	7
	1 lb	663	173.9	12
Prune Juice, canned or bottled	4 fl oz bottle	99	24.3	3
	32 fl oz bottle (1 qt)	789	194.8	21
	1 cup	197	48.6	5
	6 fl oz glass	148	36.5	4
Prune Whip, baked	1 cup served hot	140	33.2	148
	1 cup served cold	203	48.0	213
Puddings with starch base, prepared from home recipe	1 cup, chocolate	385	66.8	146
	1 cup, vanilla (blanc-mange)	283	40.5	166
Puddings, other See individual kinds: bread pudding, etc.				
Puddings made from mixes See also Pudding Mixes, brand names				
chocolate pudding made with milk, cooked	2¼ cups, yield from 4 oz mix & 2 cups milk	723	132.9	752
	1 cup	322	59.3	335
chocolate pudding made with milk, without cooking	2⅓ cups, yield from 4½ oz mix & 2 cups milk	770	150.3	764
	1 cup	325	63.4	322
Pudding Mixes, brand names Jell-O Instant Pudding & Pie Filling				
French Vanilla	½ cup pudding made with milk	160	28	440
Lemon	½ cup pudding made with milk	170	29	395
Milk Chocolate	½ cup pudding made with milk	180	30	505
Pistachio	½ cup pudding made with milk	170	28	440
Royal Pudding & Pie Filling				
Dark & Sweet Chocolate	½ cup prepared	180	33	150
Vanilla	½ cup prepared	160	27	205

Food	Quantity or Portion	Calories	Carbo-hydrates (grams)	Sodium (milli-grams)
Pudding Pops				
See Frozen Desserts				
Pumpkin, canned	1 lb can	150	35.8	9
	1 cup	81	19.4	5
Pumpkin & Squash seeds	1 cup	774	21.0	—
(kernels), dry, hulled	1 lb	2,508	68.0	—
Pumpkin Pie Spice	1 tsp	6	1.17	1

R

Food	Quantity or Portion	Calories	Carbo-hydrates (grams)	Sodium (milli-grams)
Rabbit, domesticated, flesh only, cooked (stewed)	8.6 oz, yield from 1 lb ready-to-cook rabbit	529	0	100
	1 lb	980	0	186
Radishes, raw				
whole, prepackaged without	10 lg (1 to 1¼″ diam)	14	2.9	15
tops (round, red type)	10 med (¾ to 1″ diam)	8	1.6	8
	1 cup sliced	20	4.1	21
	6 oz pkg	26	5.5	28
	1 lb	77	16.3	82
Raisins, natural (unbleached), seedless type, whole	15 oz pkg (approx 3 cups not packed)	1,228	329.0	115
	1½ oz pkg (approx ⅓ cup not packed)	124	33.3	12
	1 cup not packed	419	112.2	39
	1 cup packed	477	127.7	45
cooked seedless raisins & liquid, added sugar	1 cup	628	166.4	38
Raspberries				
fresh				
black	1 cup	98	21.0	1
	1 lb	331	71.2	5
red	1 cup	70	16.7	1
	1 lb	259	61.7	5
canned, red, water pack, berries	1 cup	85	21.4	2
& liquid, unsweetened	1 lb	159	39.9	5
frozen, red, sweetened with nu-	10 oz container	278	69.9	3
tritive sweetener, not thawed	1 cup	245	61.5	3
Redfish				
See Ocean Perch, Atlantic				
Rennin products				
tablet (salts, starch, rennin en-	12 tablets (1 pkg)	12	2.7	2,453
zyme), ⅝″ diam, ⅛″ thick	1 tablet	1	.2	201
dessert, home prepared with	2⅛ cups, yield from			
tablet	recipe	485	63.2	447
	1 cup	227	29.6	209

Food	Quantity or Portion	Calories	Carbo-hydrates (grams)	Sodium (milli-grams)
desserts prepared from mixes (prepared with milk)				
chocolate	2⅛ cups (yield from 2 oz mix & 2 cups milk)	556	77	283
	1 cup	260	36	133
vanilla, caramel or fruit dessert	2⅛ cup (yield from 1½ oz mix & 2 cups milk)	504	67.8	244
	1 cup	238	32.0	115
Rhubarb				
raw	1 lb trimmed	62	14.4	8
	1 cup diced	20	4.5	2
cooked, added sugar	1 cup	381	97.2	5
frozen, sweetened				
cooked, added sugar	1¼ cups (yield from 10 oz frozen)	486	123.1	10
	2 cups (yield from 1 lb frozen)	778	196.9	16
	1 cup	386	97.7	8
Rice, brown				
raw	1 cup long grain	666	143.2	17
	1 cup short grain	720	154.8	18
	1 lb	1,633	351.1	41
cooked, long grain (cooked with salt)	1 cup hot rice	232	49.7	550
	1 cup cold rice	173	37.0	409
	1 lb	540	115.7	1,279
Rice, white (fully milled or polished), enriched or unenriched				
raw	1 cup long grain	672	148.7	9
	1 cup med grain	708	156.8	10
	1 cup short grain	726	160.8	10
	1 lb	1,647	364.7	23
cooked (moist, soft stage), long grain (cooked with salt)	1 cup hot rice	223	49.6	767
	1 cup cold rice	158	35.1	542
	1 lb	494	109.8	1,696
parboiled, long grain, regular				
dry form	1 cup	683	150.4	17
	1 lb	1,674	368.8	41
cooked (with salt)	1 cup hot rice	186	40.8	627
	1 cup cold rice	154	33.8	519
	1 lb	481	105.7	1,624
precooked (instant), long grain				
dry form	1 cup	355	78.4	1
	1 lb	1,696	374.2	5
prepared ready to serve, fluffed	1 cup hot rice	180	39.9	450
	1 cup cold rice	142	31.5	355
	1 lb	494	109.8	1,238
Rice Mixes, brand names				
Rice A Roni				
Beef Flavor	1.3 oz, dry	130	26	780
Chicken Flavor	1.3 oz, dry	130	27	800
Spanish	1.07 oz, dry	110	22.9	720

Food	Quantity or Portion	Calories	Carbo-hydrates (grams)	Sodium (milli-grams)
Uncle Ben's				
Brown & Wild Rice	½ cup	130	25	470
Long Grain & Wild	½ cup	100	21	400
Select Brown	⅔ cup	140	29	5
Rice Polish				
stirred, spooned into cup	1 cup	278	60.6	trace
	1 lb	1,202	261.7	trace
Rice products used mainly as hot breakfast cereals (rice, granulated, with added nutrients)				
dry form	1 cup	651	146.0	—
	1 lb	1,737	389.6	—
cooked	1 cup	123	27.4	431
	1 lb	227	50.8	798
Rice-based breakfast cereals	1 cup rice, oven popped, sugar and salt added iron, vitamins	117	26.3	283
	1 cup rice, puffed, no added sugar or salt	60	13.4	trace
with presweetened rice	1 cup, oven popped, added salt, iron, vitamins	175	40.8	318
	1 cup puffed, added honey or cocoa, salt & fat, iron, vitamins	140	30.3	148
	1 cup shredded, added sugar & salt, iron, thiamine, niacin	98	22.2	229
Rice Pudding with raisins	1 cup	387	70.8	188
Rockfish, oven steamed	13 oz (yield from 1 lb raw fillets)	396	7.0	252
	1 fillet, 7 × 3⅜ × ⅝"	123	2.2	78
	1 lb	485	8.6	308
	1 oz	30	.5	19
Roe, herring, canned, solids & liquid	8 oz can	268	.7	—
	15 oz can	502	1.3	—
	1 lb	535	1.4	—
Rolls & Buns				
See also Rolls & Buns, refrigerated & ready to heat, brand names				
home baked rolls made with milk & enriched flour	1 cloverleaf roll, 2½" diam, 2" high	119	19.6	98
	1 lb, approx 13 rolls	1,538	254.5	1,266
commercial, ready-to-serve				
Danish pastry (plain without fruit or nuts)				
prepackaged ring	12 oz ring	1,435	155.0	1,244
	1 piece, ⅛ pkg	179	19.4	156

Food	Quantity or Portion	Calories	Carbo-hydrates (grams)	Sodium (milli-grams)
	5 oz round piece, approx 7″ diam	599	64.8	520
	1 piece, approx 5½″ arc, ¼ pkg	150	16.2	130
other styles	1 rectangular piece pastry, approx 6½″ long, 2¾″ wide & ¾″ high	317	34.2	275
	1 round piece pastry, approx 4¼″ diam, 1″ high	274	29.6	238
	1 lb	1,914	206.8	1,660
	1 oz	120	12.9	104
Hard rolls (enriched or unenriched)	1 roll (round or kaiser, 3¾″ diam, 2″ high; or rectangular 4¾ × 2¾ × 2½″)	156	29.8	313
	1 small rectangular roll, 3¾ × 2½ × 1¾″	78	14.9	156
	1 lb, approx 9 rolls	1,415	269.9	2,835
Hoagie or submarine roll See Bread & Rolls, French or Vienna enriched or unenriched				
plain (soft rolls or buns) (enriched or unenriched)	1 small cloverleaf roll (2½″ diam, 2″ high) or 1 small pan or dinner roll (2″ sq, 2″ high)	83	14.8	142
frankfurter (hotdog) & hamburger (sandwich)	11½ oz pkg, 8 rolls	969	172.3	1,645
	1 roll or bun	119	21.2	202
partially baked (brown-and-serve)				
enriched or unenriched, cloverleaf & pan	12 oz pkg or 12 rolls	1,017	172.0	1,649
	1 roll (1 oz)	84	14.2	136
Rolls & Buns, refrigerated & ready to heat, brand names				
Pillsbury Best				
Apple Danish	1 roll	240	33	260
Big Country Biscuits	2 biscuits	200	29	650
Caramel Danish Rolls	2 rolls	310	39	490
Cinnamon Raisin	2 rolls	290	39	450
French Loaf	1″ slice	60	11	120
Heat 'N Eat Biscuits	2 biscuits	170	27	530
Orange Flavor Danish	2 rolls	290	39	490
Quick Cinnamon rolls	1 roll	210	29	260
Hungry Jack (Pillsbury)				
Butter Tastin'	2 biscuits	180	23	310
Buttermilk Fluffy	2 biscuits	180	24	560
Sun-Maid Raisin Cinnamon Rolls	1 roll	120	17	220
Rolls, parkerhouse, baked from frozen dough	16 rolls (yield from 1 lb frozen dough)	1,216	215.0	2,059
	1 roll	75	13.3	127

Food	Quantity or Portion	Calories	Carbo-hydrates (grams)	Sodium (milli-grams)
Rolls prepared with roll mix & water, baked	1 cloverleaf roll, 2½" diam, 2" high	105	19.1	110
	1 lb, approx 13 rolls	1,356	247.2	1,420
Root Beer				
See Beverages				
Rosemary, dried	1 tsp	4	0.77	1
Roy Rogers				
Breakfast Crescent Sandwich				
Plain	127g	401	25.3	867
With Bacon	133g	431	25.5	1,035
With Ham	165g	557	25.3	1,192
With Sausage	162g	449	25.9	1,289
Crescent Roll	70g	287	27.2	547
Burgers				
Bacon Cheeseburger	180g	581	25.0	1,535
Cheeseburger	173g	563	27.4	1,404
Hamburger	143g	456	26.6	495
RR Bar Burger	208g	611	28.0	1,826
Danish				
Apple	71g	249	31.6	255
Cheese	71g	254	31.4	11
Cherry	71g	254	31.4	260
Chicken				
Breast	126g	324	7.3	601
Breast & Wing	169g	466	10.5	867
Leg	47g	117	2.1	162
Thigh	98g	282	6.5	505
Thigh & Leg	146g	399	8.6	667
Wing	43g	142	3.2	266
Egg and Biscuit Platter				
Plain	165g	394	21.9	734
With Bacon	173g	435	22.1	957
With Ham	200g	442	22.5	1,156
With Sausage	203g	550	21.9	1,059
Shakes				
Chocolate	318g	358	61.3	290
Strawberry	312g	315	49.4	261
Vanilla	306g	306	45.0	282
Sundaes				
Caramel	145g	293	51.5	193.2
Hot Fudge	151g	337	53.3	186
Strawberry	142g	216	33.1	99
Pancake Platter (with syrup & butter)	165g	452	71.8	842
With Bacon	173g	493	72.0	1,065
With Ham	200g	506	72.4	1,264
With Sausage	203g	608	71.8	1,167
Potato, Hot Topped				
Plain	227g	211	47.9	65.3
With Oleo	236g	274	47.9	161
With Bacon 'N Cheese	248g	397	33.3	778
With Broccoli 'N Cheese	312g	376	39.6	523

Food	Quantity or Portion	Calories	Carbo-hydrates (grams)	Sodium (milli-grams)
With Sour Cream 'N Chives	297g	408	47.6	138
With Taco Beef 'N Cheese	359g	463	45.0	726
Miscellaneous				
Biscuit	63g	231	26.2	575
Cole Slaw	99g	110	11.0	261
French Fries	85g	268	32.0	165
French Fries (large)	113g	357	42.7	220.5
Macaroni	110g	186	19.4	603
Potato Salad	100g	107	10.9	696
Rum				
See Beverages				
Rusk, 3⅜″ diam, ½″ thick	4 oz pkg, 13 rusks	473	80.2	278
	1 rusk	38	6.4	22
	1 lb, approx 50 rusks	1,901	322.1	1,116
Rutabagas	1 cup raw, cubed	64	15.4	7
	1 cup cooked, cubed or sliced	60	13.9	7
	1 cup cooked, mashed	84	19.7	10
	1 lb	159	37.2	18
Rye flours				
light	1 cup unsifted, spooned into cup	364	79.5	1
	1 cup sifted, spooned into cup	314	68.6	1
med	1 cup sifted, spooned into cup	308	65.8	1
dark	1 cup spooned into cup	419	87.2	1
Rye Wafers, whole grain	8 oz pkg (36 wafers, 3½″ long, 1⅞″ wide, ¼″ thick)	781	173.2	2,002
	10 wafers	224	49.6	573
	1 wafer	22	5	57

S

Food	Quantity or Portion	Calories	Carbo-hydrates (grams)	Sodium (milli-grams)
Safflower oil				
See Oils				
Saffron	1 tsp	2	0.46	1
Sage, ground	1 tsp	2	0.43	trace
Saint John's bread				
See Carob Flour				
Salad dressings, commercial				
See also Salad Dressings, brand names				
Blue & Roquefort cheese				
regular	1 cup	1,235	18.1	2,680
	1 tbsp	76	1.1	164

Food	Quantity or Portion	Calories	Carbo-hydrates (grams)	Sodium (milli-grams)
low calorie (approx 5 calories per tsp)	1 cup	194	10.5	2,825
	1 tbsp	12	.7	177
low calorie (approx 1 calorie per tsp)	1 cup	47	3.4	2,778
	1 tbsp	3	.2	170
French				
regular	1 cup	1,025	43.8	3,425
	1 tbsp	66	2.8	219
low calorie (approx 5 calories per tsp)	1 cup	250	40.6	2,046
	1 tbsp	15	2.5	126
Italian				
regular	1 cup	1,297	16.2	4,916
	1 tbsp	83	1.0	314
low calorie (approx 3 calories per tsp)	1 cup	120	6.2	1,889
	1 tbsp	8	.4	118
Mayonnaise	1 cup	1,580	4.8	1,313
	1 tbsp	101	.3	84
Russian	1 cup	1,210	25.5	2,127
	1 tbsp	74	1.6	130
salad dressing (mayonnaise type)				
regular	1 cup	1,022	33.8	1,377
	1 tbsp	65	2.2	88
low calorie (approx 8 calories per tsp)	1 cup	340	12.0	295
	1 tbsp	22	.8	19
Thousand Island				
regular	1 cup	1,255	38.5	1,750
	1 tbsp	80	2.5	112
low calorie (approx 10 calories per tsp)	1 cup	441	38.2	1,715
	1 tbsp	27	2.3	105
Salad Dressings, brand names				
Hellmann's				
Real Mayonnaise	1 tbsp	100	0	80
Relish Sandwich Spread	1 tbsp	50	2	170
Tartar Sauce	1 tbsp	70	1	140
Kraft				
Light Mayonnaise	1 tbsp	45	1	90
Real Mayonnaise	1 tbsp	100	0	70
Miracle Whip	1 tbsp	70	2	85
Miracle Whip, Light	1 tbsp	45	2	95
Weight Watchers				
Low Sodium Mayonnaise	1 tbsp	40	1	35
Regular Mayonnaise	1 tbsp	40	1	80
Whipped Salad Dressing	1 tbsp	35	3	80
Salad Oil				
See Oils				
Salami				
See Sausage, cold cuts & luncheon meats				

Food	Quantity or Portion	Calories	Carbo-hydrates (grams)	Sodium (milli-grams)
Salmon, canned, fish & liquid				
See also Salmon, brand name				
Atlantic	7¾ oz can	447	0	v
	1 lb can	921	0	v
Chinook	7¾ oz can	462	0	v
	1 lb can	953	0	v
Chum	7¾ oz can	306	0	v
	1 lb can	631	0	v
Coho (silver)	7¾ oz can	337	0	772
	1 lb can	694	0	1,592
Pink (humpback)	7¾ oz can	310	0	851
	1 lb can	640	0	1,755
Sockeye	7¾ oz can	376	0	1,148
	1 lb can	776	0	2,368
Salmon, canned, brand name				
Bumblebee				
Blueback	3.5 oz (approx ½ cup)	180	0	(a)
Pink	3.5 oz (approx ½ cup)	160	0	490
Red	3.5 oz (approx ½ cup)	180	0	(a)
Salmon steak, fresh, broiled or baked with butter or margarine (no salt added)	1 piece, 6¾″ long, 2½″ wide, 1″ thick (un-cooked dimensions) 5 oz	232	0	148
	1 lb (not fillet)	727	0	463
	1 lb fillet	826	0	526
	1 oz	52	0	33
Salmon, Smoked	1 lb	798	0	v
	1 oz	50	0	v
Salsify, cooked (boiled), drained	1 cup, cubed	(b)	20.4	—
	1 lb	(b)	68.5	—
Salt, table	1 cup	0	0	112,398
	1 tbsp	0	0	6,589
	1 tsp	0	0	2,132
Salt Sticks				
regular type (bread sticks with-out salt coating)	1 stick, 4¼″ long, ½″ diam	38	8	70
	1 stick, 7¾″ long, ¾″ diam	19	4	35
Vienna bread type	1 stick, 6½″ long, 1¼″ wide	106	20.3	548
Sandwich spread (with chopped pickle)				
regular	1 cup	929	39.0	1,534
	1 tbsp	57	2.4	94
special dietary (low calorie, ap-prox 5 calories per tsp)	1 tbsp	17	1.2	94

(a) Content not available.

(b) Values for 1 cup range from 16 calories when prepared from freshly harvested salsify to 94 calories when prepared from stored salsify. The corresponding per lb range is 54–318 calories.

Food	Quantity or Portion	Calories	Carbo-hydrates (grams)	Sodium (milli-grams)
Sardines, Atlantic, canned in oil				
sardines & oil	3¾ oz can	330	.6	541
	1 oz	88	.2	145
drained sardines only	3¾ oz can	187	v	757
	1 fish, 3½" long	41	v	165
	1 fish, 3" long	24	v	99
	1 fish, 2⅔" long, 16–20 per can	10	v	41
	1 oz	58	v	233
Sauerkraut, canned solids & liquid	1 lb can	82	18.1	3,388
	1 cup	42	9	1,755
Sauerkraut Juice, canned	15 fl oz can	45	10.4	3,565
Sausage, cold cuts & luncheon meats				
Blood sausage (blood pudding) & blood & tongue sausage	1 lb	1,787	1.4	v
	4 oz	448	0.4	v
	1 oz	112	.1	v
Bockwurst	1 link	172	.4	v
	1 lb, approx 7 links	1,198	2.7	v
Bologna, average of all types	1 lb	1,379	5.0	5,897
	4 oz	345	1.3	1,476
	1 oz	86	.3	369
Bologna, without binders	1 lb pkg	1,256	16.8	v
	4 oz	314	4.2	v
	1 oz	79	1.0	v
Bologna, with cereal	1 lb	1,188	17.7	v
	4 oz	297	4.4	v
	1 oz	74	1.1	v
Braunschweiger (smoked liverwurst)				
prepackaged forms, rolls	1 lb pkg	1,447	10.4	v
	1 slice, 2½" diam, ¼" thick, 1/25 roll	57	.4	v
	8 oz pkg	724	5.2	v
	1 slice, approx 2" diam, ¼" thick, 1/22 roll	32	.2	v
	4 oz	362	2.6	v
	1 oz	90	0.7	v
Brown-and-serve sausage				
browned	8–9 patties, or 10–11 links, yield from 8 oz pkg	760	5.0	v
	yield from ¼ lb (4 oz)	380	2.5	v
	1 patty	97	.6	v
	1 link	72	.5	v
Capicola or Cappacola	1 lb	2,263	0	v
	4 oz	566	0	v
	1 oz	141	0	v
Cervelat, dry	1 lb	2,046	7.7	v
	4 oz	512	2	v
	1 oz	128	.5	v

Food	Quantity or Portion	Calories	Carbo-hydrates (grams)	Sodium (milli-grams)
Cervelat, soft See Thuringer Cervelat (summer sausage)				
Country-style sausage	1 lb	1,565	0	v
	4 oz	391	0	v
Deviled ham, canned	2¼ oz can	225	0	v
	3 oz can	298	0	v
	4½ oz can	449	0	v
	1 cup	790	0	v
	1 tbsp	46	0	v
	1 lb	1,592	0	v
	4 oz	398	0	v
	1 oz	100	0	v
Frankfurters (franks, hotdogs, wieners)				
prepackaged frankfurters, average of all types	1 lb pkg, approx 8–10 frankfurters	1,402	8.2	4,990
	1 frankfurter, approx 5″ long, ⅞″ diam, 2 oz (8 per lb)	176	1.0	627
	1 frankfurter, 5″ long, ¾″ diam, 1.6 oz (10 per lb)	139	.8	495
without binders not smoked	1 lb pkg, 8–10 frankfurters	1,343	11.3	v
	1 frankfurter, approx 5″ long, ⅞″ diam, 2 oz (8 per lb)	169	1.4	v
	1 frankfurter, 5″ long, ¾″ diam, 1.6 oz (10 per lb)	133	1.1	v
	1 cocktail frank, 1¾″ long, ½″ diam, ⅓ oz	30	.3	v
smoked	12 oz pkg, 8–10 frankfurters	1,006	8.5	v
	1 frankfurter, approx 4¾″ long, ¾″ diam, 1½ oz	124	1.1	v
	1 frankfurter, 4½″ long, ¾″ diam, 1.2 oz (10 per pkg)	101	.9	v
	1 cocktail frank, 1¾″ long, ⅝″ diam, ⅓ oz	27	.2	v
made with cereal	1 lb pkg, 8–10 frankfurters	1,125	.9	v
	1 frankfurter, approx 5″ long, ⅞″ diam, 2 oz	141	.1	v
	1 frankfurter, 5″ long, ¾″ diam, 1.6 oz	112	.1	v

Food	Quantity or Portion	Calories	Carbo-hydrates (grams)	Sodium (milli-grams)
canned frankfurters	7 frankfurters, drained contents 12 oz can	751	.7	v
	1 frankfurter, 4⅞″ long, ⅞″ diam, 1½ oz	106	.1	v
	1 lb	1,002	.9	v
Headcheese	1 lb	1,216	4.5	v
	4 oz	304	1.1	v
	1 oz slice	76	.3	v
Knockwurst				
prepackaged links, approx 4″ long, 1⅛″ diam, 2.4 oz each	12 oz pkg, approx 5 links	945	7.5	v
	1 link	189	1.5	v
	1 lb	1,261	10.0	v
	4 oz	315	2.5	v
Liverwurst				
fresh (not smoked)	1 lb	1,393	8.2	v
	4 oz	348	2.0	v
	1 oz	87	.5	v
smoked See Braunschweiger				
Luncheon meat				
boiled ham base	8 oz pkg	531	0	v
	6 oz pkg	398	0	v
	1 lb	1,061	0	v
	4 oz	265	0	v
	1 oz	66	0	v
pork, cured ham or shoulder base, chopped, canned	12 oz can	1,000	4.4	4,196
	7 oz can	582	2.6	2,443
	1 lb	1,334	5.9	5,597
	4 oz	334	1.5	1,399
	1 oz	83	.4	350
Meatloaf	1 lb	907	15.0	v
	4 oz	227	3.8	v
	1 oz	57	.9	v
Meat, potted (includes potted beef, chicken, turkey)	3–3¼ oz can	223	0	v
	5½ oz can	387	0	v
	1 cup	558	0	v
	1 tbsp	32	0	v
	1 lb	1,125	0	v
	4 oz	281	0	v
	1 oz	70	0	v
Minced ham	1 lb	1,034	20.0	v
	4 oz	258	5.0	v
Mortadella	1 lb	1,429	2.7	v
	4 oz	357	.7	v
	1 oz	89	.2	v
Polish sausage				
prepackaged links	1 lb pkg	1,379	5.4	v
	1 sausage, 10″ long, 1¼″ diam, 8 oz	690	2.7	v

Food	Quantity or Portion	Calories	Carbo-hydrates (grams)	Sodium (milli-grams)
	1 sausage, 5⅜" long, 1" diam, 2.7 oz	231	.9	v
	4 oz	345	1.4	v
	1 oz	86	.3	v
Pork sausage cooked	7½ oz, yield from 1 lb, raw	1,014	trace	2,041
	3.8 oz, yield from 8 oz raw	509	trace	1,025
	1.9 oz, yield from 4 oz raw	254	trace	510
	1 piece, 3" long, 1¼" diam, 2.4 oz, raw	152	trace	307
	1 patty, 3⅞" diam, ¼" thick, 2 oz, raw	129	trace	259
	1 link, 4" long, ⅞" diam, 1 oz, raw	62	trace	125
canned, sausage & liquid	8 oz can, approx 14 links	942	5.4	v
drained sausage	8 oz can, approx 14 links	617	3.1	v
	1 link	46	.2	v
	1 lb dry	1,728	8.6	v
	1 oz dry	108	.5	v
Pork sausage, link, smoked See Sausage, country-style Salami				
dry, prepackaged roll	8 oz roll, approx 6⅝" long, 1¾" diam	1,053	2.8	v
	1 lb	2,041	5.4	v
	4 oz	510	1.4	v
	1 oz	128	.3	v
cooked, prepackaged slices	1 lb	1,411	6.4	v
	4 oz	353	1.6	v
	1 oz	88	.4	v
Scrapple, prepackaged loaf	1 lb	975	66.2	v
	4 oz	244	16.6	v
	1 oz	61	4.1	v
Souse	1 lb	821	5.4	v
	4 oz	205	1.4	v
	1 oz	51	.3	v
Thuringer cervelat (summer sausage)	1 lb	1,393	7.3	v
	4 oz	348	1.8	v
	1 oz	87	.5	v
Vienna sausage, canned	7 sausages, contents of 5 oz can	271	.3	v
	1 sausage	38	trace	v
Savory, ground	1 tsp	4	0.96	trace
Scallions (young green onions) bulb and white portion of top	2 med (4⅛" long, ⅝" diam) or 6 small			

Food	Quantity or Portion	Calories	Carbo-hydrates (grams)	Sodium (milli-grams)
	scallions (3″ long, ⅜″ diam)	14	3.2	2
	1 cup chopped or sliced	45	10.5	5
	1 tbsp chopped	3	.6	trace
	1 lb	204	47.6	23
tops only (green portion)	1 cup	27	5.5	5
	1 tbsp chopped	2	.3	trace
	1 lb	122	24.9	23
Scallops, bay and sea				
cooked (steamed)	1 lb	508	—	1,202
frozen, breaded, fried, reheated (sea scallops)	6⅔ oz (yield from 7 oz container, 15–20 scallops)	367	19.8	—
	11.4 oz (yield from 12 oz container, 30–35 scallops)	629	34.0	—
	1 lg scallop, 15–20 per lb	49	2.6	—
	1 med scallop, 25–30 per lb	29	1.6	—
Scrapple				
See Sausage, cold cuts & luncheon meats				
Sesame Oil				
See Oils				
Sesame seeds, dry, hulled, decorticated	1 cup	873	26.4	—
	1 tbsp	47	1.4	—
Shad, baked	12⅞ oz, yield from 1 lb raw fillets	734	0	288
	1 lb	912	0	358
	1 oz	57	0	22
Shallot bulbs, raw, chopped	1 tbsp	7	1.7	1
Sherbet, orange	½ gal prepackaged container	2,066	474.9	154
	1 cup, 8 fl oz	259	59.4	19
Shrimp				
cooked (french fried)	1 lb	1,021	45.4	844
	1 oz	64	2.8	53
canned				
drained shrimp from wet pack	4½ oz can, approx 1 cup, 22 lg, 40 med, or 76 small shrimp	148	.9	—
	10 large shrimp, approx 3¼″ long	67	0.4	—
	10 med shrimp, approx 2½″ long	37	.2	—
	10 small shrimp, approx 2″ long	20	.1	—
	1 lb	526	3.2	—
	1 oz	33	.2	—

Food	Quantity or Portion	Calories	Carbo-hydrates (grams)	Sodium (milli-grams)
Shrimp or lobster paste, canned	1 tsp	13	.1	—
Snacks, name brands				
Bachman Jax	1 oz	150	17	340
Bugles				
Regular	1 oz	150	18	290
Nacho Cheese	1 oz	160	17	270
Chee-Tos Puffs	1 oz	160	15	370
Doritos Tortilla Chips				
Nacho Cheese	1 oz	140	18	250
Taco	1 oz	140	18	280
Fritos Original Corn Chips	1 oz	150	16	230
Herr's				
Bar-B-Q Flavor Corn Chips	1 oz	150	16	280
Corn Chips	1 oz	150	16	160
Nacho Cheese Tortilla Chips	1 oz	130	20	180
Toasted Tortilla Chips	1 oz	140	17	250
Tostitos				
Nacho Cheese	1 oz	150	17	220
Traditional	1 oz	140	18	180
Soft Drinks				
See Beverages				
Soups				
See also, Soups, brand names				
Soups, canned				
Asparagus, cream of				
condensed	10½ oz can	161	25.0	2,444
	1 cup	132	20.6	2,009
prepared with equal volume water	1 cup	65	10.1	984
prepared with equal volume milk	1 cup	147	16.7	1,068
Bean with pork				
condensed	10½ oz can	437	56.4	2,628
	1 cup	355	45.8	2,136
prepared with equal volume water	1 cup	168	21.8	1,008
Beef broth, bouillon or con-somme				
condensed	10½ oz can	77	6.6	1,943
	1 cup	64	5.4	1,597
prepared with equal voume water	1 cup	31	2.6	782
Beef noodle				
condensed	10½ oz can	170	17.3	2,277
	1 cup	140	14.2	1,872
prepared with equal volume water	1 cup	67	7.0	917
Celery, cream of				
condensed	10½ oz can	215	22.1	2,372
	1 cup	176	18.1	1,950

Food	Quantity or Portion	Calories	Carbo-hydrates (grams)	Sodium (milli-grams)
prepared with equal volume water	1 cup	86	8.9	955
prepared with equal volume milk	1 cup	169	15.2	1,039
Chicken consomme				
condensed	10½ oz can	54	4.5	1,794
	1 cup	44	3.7	1,475
prepared with equal volume water	1 cup	22	1.9	722
Chicken, cream of				
condensed	10½ oz can	235	20.0	2,411
	1 cup	194	16.4	1,982
prepared with equal volume water	1 cup	94	7.9	970
prepared with equal volume milk	1 cup	179	14.5	1,054
Chicken gumbo				
condensed	10½ oz can	137	18.2	2,360
	1 cup	113	14.9	1,940
prepared with equal volume water	1 cup	55	7.4	950
Chicken noodle				
condensed	10½ oz can	158	19.7	2,432
	1 cup	130	16.2	1,999
prepared with equal volume water	1 cup	62	7.9	979
Chicken with rice				
condensed	10½ oz can	116	14.0	2,277
	1 cup	96	11.5	1,872
prepared with equal volume water	1 cup	48	5.8	917
Chicken vegetable				
condensed	10½ oz can	187	23.3	2,552
	1 cup	155	19.3	2,113
prepared with equal volume water	1 cup	76	9.6	1,034
Clam chowder, Manhattan type (with tomatoes, without milk)				
condensed	10½ oz can	201	30.5	2,336
	1 cup	165	25.0	1,915
prepared with equal volume of water	1 cup	81	12.3	938
Minestrone				
condensed	10½ oz can	265	35.4	2,480
	1 cup	218	29.0	2,033
prepared with equal volume water	1 cup	105	14.2	995
Mushroom, cream of				
condensed	10½ oz can	331	25.0	2,369
	1 cup	272	20.6	1,948

Food	Quantity or Portion	Calories	Carbo-hydrates (grams)	Sodium (milli-grams)
prepared with equal volume water	1 cup	134	10.1	955
prepared with equal volume milk	1 cup	216	16.2	1,039
Onion				
condensed	10½ oz can	161	12.8	2,608
	1 cup	132	10.5	2,144
prepared with equal volume water	1 cup	65	5.3	1,051
Pea, green				
condensed	10½ oz can	335	58.1	2,319
	1 cup	270	46.9	1,872
prepared with equal volume water	1 cup	130	22.5	899
prepared with equal volume milk	1 cup	213	29.3	983
Pea, split				
condensed	10½ oz can	376	54.2	2,447
	1 cup	301	43.4	1,956
prepared with equal volume of water	1 cup	145	20.6	941
Tomato				
condensed	10½ oz can	220	38.7	2,416
	1 cup	180	31.8	1,980
prepared with equal volume water	1 cup	88	15.7	970
prepared with equal volume of milk	1 cup	173	22.5	1,055
Turkey noodle				
condensed	10½ oz can	194	20.9	2,479
	1 cup	159	17.2	2,038
prepared with equal volume water	1 cup	79	8.4	998
Vegetable beef				
condensed	10½ oz can	198	24.1	2,605
	1 cup	163	19.8	2,135
prepared with equal volume water	1 cup	78	9.6	1,046
Vegetable with beef broth				
condensed	10½ oz can	195	33.6	2,105
	1 cup	160	27.5	1,725
prepared with equal volume water	1 cup	78	13.5	845
Vegetarian vegetable				
condensed	10½ oz can	195	32.3	2,086
	1 cup	160	26.5	1,710
prepared with equal volume water	1 cup	78	13.2	838
Soups, dehydrated				
Beef noodle	1 pkg mix, dry form (2 oz pkg)	221	37.2	1,350

Food	Quantity or Portion	Calories	Carbo-hydrates (grams)	Sodium (milli-grams)
Chicken noodle	1 cup prepared with 2 oz mix in 3 cups water	67	11.5	420
	1 pkg mix, dry form (2 oz pkg)	218	33.1	2,438
Chicken rice	1 cup prepared with 2 oz mix in 4 cups water	53	7.7	578
	1 pkg mix, dry form (1½ oz pkg)	152	27.0	1,876
Onion	1 cup prepared with 1½ oz mix in 3 cups water	48	8.4	622
	1 pkg mix, dry form (1½ oz pkg)	150	23.2	2,871
Pea, green	1 cup prepared with 1½ oz mix in 4 cups water	36	5.5	689
	1 pkg mix, dry form (4 oz pkg)	409	69.6	2,667
Tomato vegetable with noodles	1 cup prepared with 4 oz mix in 3 cups water	123	20.6	796
	1 pkg mix, dry form (2½ oz pkg)	247	44.5	4,357
	1 cup prepared with 2½ oz mix in 4 cups water	65	12.2	1,025

Soups, brand names
Campbell Soups (content for 4 oz condensed, 8 oz prepared)

Food	Quantity or Portion	Calories	Carbo-hydrates (grams)	Sodium (milli-grams)
Beef Broth (Bouillon)		16	1	860
Beef Noodle		70	7	875
Beef with Bacon		150	2	860
Cheddar Cheese, prepared with milk		130	10	800
Chicken Barley		70	10	900
Chicken Gumbo		60	8	910
Chicken Noodle		70	9	840
Chicken Vegetable		79	8	870
Clam Chowder (Manhattan)		70	11	860
Clam Chowder (New England, prepared with milk)		150	17	930
Consomme (Beef)		25	2	785
Cream of Mushroom		100	9	825
French Onion		60	9	950
Green Pea		160	25	840
Nacho Cheese (prepared with milk)		210	15	760
Oyster Stew (prepared with milk)		150	10	900
Tomato (prepared with milk)		160	22	800
Tomato Rice		110	22	760
Turkey Noodle		60	8	910

Food	Quantity or Portion	Calories	Carbo-hydrates (grams)	Sodium (milli-grams)
Vegetable, Old Fashioned		60	9	910
Vegetable, Vegetarian		70	12	755
Campbell's Creamy Natural Soups (content for 8 oz, prepared with 4 oz soup and 4 oz milk)				
Creamy Asparagus		200	13	840
Creamy Potato		220	16	860
Creamy Spinach		160	14	700
Campbell's Chunky Soups (content for 10¾ oz, ready to serve)				
Beef		190	23	1,110
Chicken		170	21	1,340
Chicken Noodle with Mushrooms		200	20	1,190
Vegetable		140	23	1,110
Campbell's Low-Sodium Soups (content for 10½ oz, ready to serve)				
Chicken Broth		40	3	100
Chunky Vegetable Beef		170	19	65
Cream of Mushroom		190	16	60
Herb-Ox Instant Broth				
Low Sodium				
Beef	1 packet	11	2	10
Chicken	1 packet	12	2	5
Lipton Soup Mixes				
Chicken Noodle	8 fl oz	70	9	820
Noodle	8 fl oz	70	10	780
Onion	8 fl oz	35	6	640
Lipton Cup-A-Soup				
Chicken Noodle	6 fl oz	50	7	690
Chicken Vegetable	6 fl oz	40	7	780
Cream of Chicken	6 fl oz	80	9	840
Cream of Mushroom	6 fl oz	80	9	830
Harvest Vegetable	6 fl oz	90	20	625
Spicy Vegetable	6 fl oz	40	7	865
Lipton Trim Cup-A-Soup				
Chicken	6 fl oz	10	1	560
Beefy Tomato	6 fl oz	10	2	440
Herb Chicken	6 fl oz	10	1	555
Herb Vegetable	6 fl oz	10	1	560
MBT				
Beef	1 packet	12	2	960
Chicken	1 packet	14	2	1,760
Soursop, raw	1 cup, pureed	146	36.7	32
	1 lb	295	73.9	64

Souse
See Sausage, cold cuts & luncheon meats

Food	Quantity or Portion	Calories	Carbo-hydrates (grams)	Sodium (milli-grams)
Soybeans				
mature seeds, dry				
raw	1 cup	846	70.4	11
	1 lb	1,828	152.0	23
cooked	1 cup	234	19.4	4
	1 lb	590	49.0	9
sprouted seeds				
raw	1 cup	48	5.6	—
	1 lb	209	24.0	—
cooked (boiled), drained	1 cup	48	4.6	—
	1 lb	172	16.8	—
Soybean curd (tofu)	1 piece, 2½ × 2¾ × 1″	86	2.9	8
	1 lb	327	10.9	32
Soybean flours				
full fat	1 cup, not stirred	358	25.8	1
	1 cup, stirred	295	21.3	1
	1 lb	1,910	137.9	5
low fat	1 cup, stirred	313	32.2	1
	1 lb	1,615	166.0	5
defatted	1 cup, stirred	326	38.1	1
	1 lb	1,479	172.8	5
Soybean Oil				
See Oils				
Soy Sauce	1 cup	197	27.6	21,243
	1 fl oz	25	3.5	2,666
	1 tbsp	12	1.7	1,319
Spaghetti (regular, thin or vermicelli)				
enriched or unenriched, cooked from dry form				
cooked, firm ("al dente")	8.8 cups (yield from 1 lb dry)	1,674	341.1	9
	4.4 cups (yield from 8 oz dry)	838	170.7	5
	1 cup	192	39.1	1
cooked, tender	10.6 cups (yield from 1 lb dry)	1,674	341.1	9
	5.3 cups (yield from 8 oz dry)	838	170.7	5
	1 cup	155	32.2	1
Spaghetti (enriched) in tomato sauce with cheese				
cooked from home recipe	1 cup	260	37.0	955
	1 lb	472	67.1	1,733
canned	15¼ oz can	328	66.5	1,650
	1 cup	190	38.5	955
	1 lb	345	69.9	1,733
Spaghetti (enriched) with meatballs & tomato sauce				
cooked from home recipe	1 cup	332	38.6	1,009

Food	Quantity or Portion	Calories	Carbo-hydrates (grams)	Sodium (milli-grams)
	1 lb	608	70.8	1,846
	1 portion, 2⅙ cups of mixture of spaghetti, meatballs, tomato sauce; 2 tbsp grated parmesan cheese as topping	720	83.8	2,186
canned	15 oz can	438	48.5	2,074
	1 cup	258	28.5	1,220
	1 lb	467	51.7	2,214
Spaghetti, canned, brand name				
Spaghetti-O's				
In Tomato & Cheese Sauce	7⅜ oz	170	34	910
With Meatballs	7⅜ oz	220	28	910
With Sliced Beef Franks	7⅜ oz	220	26	1,070
Spaghetti Frozen Dinners				
See Frozen, Dinners, brand name				
Spanish Rice, cooked from home recipe	1 cup	213	40.7	774
Spinach				
raw, prepackaged	10 oz container	74	12.2	202
	1 cup, chopped	14	2.4	39
	1 lb	118	19.5	322
cooked (boiled), drained	1 cup leaves	41	6.5	90
	1 lb	104	16.3	227
canned, whole leaf, cut leaf or chopped				
regular pack				
spinach & liquid	7¾ oz can	42	6.6	519
	15 oz can	81	12.8	1,003
	1 cup	44	7.0	548
drained spinach	5¼ oz can	36	5.4	352
	10¼ oz can	70	10.5	687
	1 cup	49	7.4	484
	1 lb	109	16.3	1,070
special dietary pack (low sodium)				
spinach & liquid	7¾ oz can	46	7.3	75
	15 oz can	89	14.0	145
	1 cup	49	7.7	794
	1 lb	95	15.0	154
drained spinach	5¼ oz can	39	6.0	48
	10¼ oz can	76	11.6	93
	1 cup	53	8.2	66
	1 lb	118	18.1	145
frozen, chopped—cooked (boiled), drained	1¹⁄₁₆ cups, yield from 10 oz frozen	51	8.1	114
	1.7 cups, yield from 1 lb frozen	81	13.0	182
	1 cup	47	7.6	107

Food	Quantity or Portion	Calories	Carbo-hydrates (grams)	Sodium (milli-grams)
frozen, leaf—cooked (boiled), drained	1⅛ cups, yield from 10 oz frozen	53	8.6	108
	1⅞ cups, yield from 1 lb frozen	84	13.7	172
	1 cup	46	7.4	93
Spinach, New Zealand See New Zealand spinach				
Spot, baked	1 lb	1,338	0	1,415
	1 oz	84	0	88
Squash, summer				
Crookneck & Straightneck, Yellow				
raw	1 cup sliced, cubed or diced	26	5.6	1
	1 lb	91	19.5	5
cooked (boiled), drained	1 cup sliced	27	5.6	2
	1 cup cubed or diced	32	6.5	2
	1 cup mashed	36	7.4	2
	1 lb	68	14.1	5
Scallop varieties, white & pale green				
raw	1 cup sliced, cubed or diced	27	6.6	1
	1 lb	95	23.1	5
cooked (boiled), drained	1 cup sliced	29	6.8	2
	1 cup cubed or diced	34	8.0	2
	1 cup mashed	38	9.1	2
	1 lb	73	17.2	5
Zucchini & Cocozelle (Italian marrow type), green				
raw	1 cup sliced, cubed or diced	22	4.7	1
	1 lb	77	16.3	5
cooked (boiled), drained	1 cup sliced	22	4.5	2
	1 cup cubed or diced	25	5.3	2
	1 cup mashed	29	6.0	2
	1 lb	54	11.3	5
Squash, winter				
Acorn				
raw	1 whole squash, 4″ diam, 4⅓″ high, 1¼ lb (weighed whole)	190	48.3	4
baked	yield from 1 whole squash	172	43.6	4
	1 cup	113	28.7	2
	1 lb	249	63.5	5
boiled	1 cup, mashed	83	20.6	2
	1 lb	154	38.1	5

Food	Quantity or Portion	Calories	Carbo-hydrates (grams)	Sodium (milli-grams)
Butternut, cooked				
baked	1 cup	139	35.9	2
	1 lb	308	79.4	5
boiled	1 cup, mashed	100	24.5	2
	1 lb	186	47.2	5
Hubbard, cooked				
baked	1 cup	103	24.0	2
	1 lb	227	53.1	5
boiled	1 cup, cubed or diced	71	16.2	2
	1 cup, mashed	74	16.9	2
	1 lb	136	31.3	5
Squash, winter, frozen				
not thawed	12 oz container	129	31.3	3
	1 lb	172	41.7	5
cooked (heated)	1 cup	91	22.1	2
	1 lb	172	41.7	5
Starch				
See Cornstarch				
Steak Sliced, frozen, brand names				
Steak-Umm	2 oz	180	0	40
Steakwich	2 oz	160	0	40
Strawberries				
fresh	1 pt container, good quality	121	27.4	3
	1 pt container, fair quality	109	24.8	3
	1 cup whole	55	12.5	1
	1 lb	168	38.1	5
canned, water pack, berries & liquid, without artificial sweetener	1 cup	53	13.6	2
	1 lb	100	25.4	5
frozen, sweetened with nutritive sweetener, not thawed				
sliced	10 oz container	310	79.0	3
	1 lb container	494	126.1	5
	1 cup	278	70.9	3
whole	1 lb container	417	106.6	5
	1 cup	235	59.9	3
Stuffing Mix, brand names				
Betty Crocker Stuffing Mix				
Chicken	½ cup	110	21	530
Traditional Herb	½ cup	110	22	560
Stove Top				
Beef	½ cup	110	22	450
Chicken	½ cup	110	20	480
Cornbread	½ cup	110	21	590
Long Grain & Wild Rice	½ cup	110	22	460
Pork	½ cup	110	20	540
Sturgeon				
cooked, steamed	1 lb	726	0	490
	1 oz	45	0	31

Food	Quantity or Portion	Calories	Carbo-hydrates (grams)	Sodium (milli-grams)
smoked	1 lb	676	0	v
	1 oz	42	0	v
Succotash (corn, & lima beans), frozen				
cooked (boiled), drained	1 cup	158	34.9	65
	1 lb	422	93.0	172
Sugars, beet or cane				
brown, spooned into cup	1 cup, not packed	541	139.8	44
	1 cup, packed	821	212.1	66
white, granulated	1 cup	770	199.0	2
	1 tbsp	46	11.9	trace
	1 tsp	15	4.0	trace
	1 tablet or lump or 2 cubes, ½" inch	19	5.0	trace
	5–7g packet	23	6.0	trace
white, powdered (10X or confectioners)				
unsifted, spooned into cup	1 cup	462	119.4	1
	1 tbsp	31	8.0	trace
sifted, spooned into cup	1 cup	385	99.5	1
Sugar, maple (piece, approx, 1¾ × 1¼ × ½," 1 oz)	1 oz piece	99	25.5	1
Sugar Apples (sweetsop), raw, pulp	1 cup	235	59.3	28
Sunflower seed kernels, dry				
in hull	1 lb	1,371	48.7	73
	1 cup	257	9.1	14
hulled	1 lb container	2,540	90.3	136
	1 cup	812	28.9	44
Sweetbreads (thymus), cooked (braised)				
beef (yearlings)	3 oz	272	0	99
calf	3 oz	143	0	—
lamb	3 oz	149	0	—
Sweet Potatoes				
raw, weighed whole	1 lb	372	85.9	33
cooked				
baked in skin (a)	5" long, 2" diam (dimensions before cooking)	161	37.0	14
	1 lb (weighed with skins)	499	115.0	42
boiled in skin (a)	5" long, 2" diam (dimensions before cooking)	172	39.8	15
	1 lb (weighed with skins)	434	100.2	38
	1 cup, mashed	291	67.1	26
	1 lb (without skins)	517	119.3	45

(a) Calorie and other values exclude skin.

SWEET POTATOES

Food	Quantity or Portion	Calories	Carbo-hydrates (grams)	Sodium (milli-grams)
candied				
1 piece, 2½" long, 2" diam	1 piece	176	35.9	44
(dimensions before cooking), (approx ½ potato, hand peeled)	1 lb	762	155.1	191
canned				
regular pack in syrup (sweet potatoes & syrup)	1 lb	517	124.7	218
vacuum or solid pack	1 piece, 2¾" long, 1" diam	43	10.0	19
	1 cup, pieces	216	49.8	96
	1 cup, mashed	275	63.5	122
	1 lb	490	112.9	218
dehydrated flakes	1 cup dry form	455	108.0	217
	1 cup, prepared with water	242	57.6	115
	1 lb	431	102.5	204
Sweetsop				
See Sugar Apples				
Swiss Chard				
See Chard, Swiss				
Swordfish, broiled with butter or margarine	10.1 oz, yield from 1 lb raw	499	0	—
	1 piece, 4½ × 2⅛ × ⅞"	237	0	—
	1 lb	742	0	—
	1 oz	46	0	—
Syrups				
maple	12 fl oz bottle	1,189	306.8	47
	1 cup	794	204.8	32
	1 tbsp	50	12.8	2
sorghum	1 cup	848	224.4	—
	1 tbsp	53	14.0	—
table blends, chiefly corn, light & dark	16 fl oz (1 pint) bottle	1,905	492.8	447
	1 cup	951	246.0	223
	1 tbsp	59	15.4	14
table blends of cane & maple	12 fl oz bottle	1,189	306.8	9
	1 cup	794	204.8	6
	1 tbsp	50	12.8	trace
Syrup, brand names				
Aunt Jemima				
Butterlite	1 fl oz	50	13	65
Lite	1 fl oz	50	13	65
Karo				
Regular	1 tbsp	60	15	35
Dark Corn	1 tbsp	60	15	40
Light Corn	1 tbsp	60	15	30
Log Cabin Lite	1 fl oz	80	20	65

Food	Quantity or Portion	Calories	Carbo-hydrates (grams)	Sodium (milli-grams)

T

Tangelo Juice, raw, & tangelos used for juice

Food	Quantity or Portion	Calories	Carbo-hydrates (grams)	Sodium (milli-grams)
juice	1 cup	101	24.0	—
fruit used for juice	1 lg fruit, 2¾″ diam	47	11.1	—
	1 med fruit, 2⁹⁄₁₆″ diam	39	9.2	—
	1 small fruit, 2¼″ diam	28	6.6	—
Tangerines, fresh (Dancy variety)	1 lg fruit, 2½″ diam	46	11.7	2
	1 med fruit, 2⅜″ diam	39	10.0	2
	1 small fruit, 2¼″ diam	33	8.3	1
	1 cup sections, without membranes	90	22.6	4
Tangerine Juice				
fresh (Dancy variety)	1 cup	106	24.9	2
canned				
unsweetened	6 fl oz can	80	18.9	2
	1 cup	106	25.2	2
	1 fl oz	13	3.2	trace
sweetened with nutritive sweetener	6 fl oz can	94	22.4	2
	1 cup	125	29.9	2
	1 fl oz	16	3.7	trace
frozen concentrate, unsweetened undiluted	6 fl oz can (yields 3 cups diluted juice)	342	80.8	4
	12 fl oz can (yields 1½ qt diluted juice)	684	161.6	8
diluted with 3 parts water by volume	1 qt	456	107.1	10
	1 cup	114	26.8	2
	6 fl oz glasses	86	20.1	2
Tapioca, dry (pearl & granulated quick-cooking)	8 oz pkg (approx 1½ cups)	799	196.1	7
	1 cup	535	131.3	5
	1 tbsp	30	7.3	trace
Tapioca Desserts	1 cup apple tapioca	293	73.5	128
	1 cup tapioca cream pudding	221	28.2	257
Tarragon, ground	1 tsp	5	0.80	1
Tartar Sauce				
regular	1 cup	1,221	9.7	1,626
	1 tbsp	74	.6	99
special dietary (low calorie, approx 10 calories per tsp)	1 tbsp	31	.9	99
Tendergreen See Mustard spinach				
Thuringer See Sausage, cold cuts, & luncheon meats				
Thyme, ground	1 tsp	4	0.89	1
Tilefish, baked	1 lb	626	0	—
	1 oz	39	0	—

Food	Quantity or Portion	Calories	Carbo-hydrates (grams)	Sodium (milli-grams)
Tofu				
See Soybean curd				
Tofu, Frozen, brand name				
See Frozen Desserts				
Tomatoes, green, raw	1 lb	99	21.1	12
Tomatoes, ripe				
raw, not peeled	1 lb	91	19.4	12
	1 tomato, 3" diam, wt 7 oz	40	8.6	5
	1 tomato, 2.6" diam, wt 4¾ oz	27	5.8	4
	1 tomato, 2.4" diam, wt 3½ oz	20	4.3	3
cooked (boiled)	1 cup	63	13.3	10
canned, tomatoes & liquid				
regular pack	1 lb can	95	19.5	590
	28 oz can	167	34.1	1,032
	1 cup	51	10.4	313
special dietary pack (low sodium)	1 lb can	91	19.1	14
	1 cup	48	10.1	7
Tomato Catsup				
See Tomato Ketchup				
Tomato Chili sauce	12 oz bottle	354	84.3	4,549
	1 cup	284	67.7	3,653
	1 tbsp	16	3.7	201
	1 lb	472	112.5	6,069
Tomato Juice				
canned or bottled				
regular pack	1 qt bottle	185	41.8	1,944
	18 fl oz can	104	23.5	1,094
	5½ fl oz can	32	7.2	334
	1 cup	46	10.4	485
	6 fl oz glass	35	7.8	364
	1 fl oz	6	1.3	61
special dietary pack (low sodium)	18 fl oz can	104	23.4	16
	12 fl oz can	69	15.6	11
	1 cup	46	10.4	7
	6 fl oz glass	35	7.8	5
	1 fl oz	6	1.3	1
dehydrated (crystals)				
dry form	1 oz	86	19.3	1,115
	1 lb, yields approx 1¾ gal juice	1,374	309.4	17,845
	1 cup prepared with water	49	10.9	627
Tomato Juice Cocktail, canned or bottled	26 fl oz bottle (1 pt, 10 fl oz)	165	39.4	1,576
	1 cup	51	12.2	486
	6 fl oz glass	38	9.1	364
	1 fl oz	6	1.5	61

Food	Quantity or Portion	Calories	Carbo-hydrates (grams)	Sodium (milli-grams)
Tomato Ketchup	14 oz bottle	421	100.8	4,137
	20 oz (1 lb 4 oz) bottle	601	144.0	5,908
	½ oz packet	15	3.6	146
	1 cup	289	69.3	2,845
	1 tbsp	16	3.8	156
	1 lb	481	115.2	4,727
Tomato Paste, canned	6 oz can	139	31.6	65
	1 cup	215	48.7	100
	1 lb	372	84.4	172
Tomato Puree, canned				
regular pack	29 oz (1 lb 13 oz)	321	73.2	3,280
	1 lb	177	40.4	1,810
special dietary pack (low sodium)	1 lb	177	40.4	27
Tongue, cooked (braised)				
beef, med fat	1 slice, 3 × 2 × ⅛"	49	.1	12
	1 lb, approx 23 slices	1,107	1.8	277
calf	1 slice, 3 × 2 × ⅛"	32	.2	v
	1 lb, approx 23 slices	726	4.5	v
hog	1 slice, 3 × 2 × ⅛"	51	.1	v
	1 lb, approx 23 slices	1,148	2.3	v
lamb	1 slice, 3 × 2 × ⅛"	51	.1	v
	1 lb, approx 23 slices	1,152	2.3	v
sheep	1 slice, 3 × 2 × ⅛"	65	.5	v
	1 lb, approx 23 slices	1,465	10.9	v
Tuna, brand names				
Bumble Bee				
Chunk Light in Water	2 oz	70	12	310
Chunk White in Oil	2 oz	170	12	310
Solid White in Oil	2 oz	150	0	310
Solid White in Water	2 oz	70	0	310
Star-Kist				
Chunk Light in Oil	2 oz	150	1	310
Chunk Light in Water	2 oz	100	0	310
Solid White in Oil	2 oz	140	—	310
Solid White in Water	2 oz	150	1	310
Chicken of the Sea				
Chunk Light in Less Salt	2 oz	60	0	135
Chunk Light in Oil	2 oz	170	0	310
Chunk Light in Water	2 oz	60	0	310
Solid White in Oil	2 oz	120	0	310
Solid White in Water	2 oz	60	0	310
Tuna canned				
in oil				
tuna & oil	1 can, solid pack, 7 oz	570	0	1,584
	1 can, chunk style, 6½ oz	530	0	1,472
	1 can, flake or grated style, 6–6¼ oz	501	0	1,392
drained tuna	1 can, solid pack, 6 oz	333	0	v
	1 can chunk style, 5½ oz	309	0	v

Food	Quantity or Portion	Calories	Carbo-hydrates (grams)	Sodium (milli-grams)
	1 cup, solid pack or chunk style	315	0	v
	1 lb, solid pack or chunk style	894	0	v
in water				
tuna & water	1 can solid pack, 3½ oz	126	0	41
	1 can chunk style, 3⅛ oz	117	0	38
	1 can solid pack, 7 oz	251	0	81
	1 can chunk style, 6½ oz	234	0	75
	1 lb, all styles	576	0	186
Tuna Mix, brand name				
Tuna Helper	⅕ pkg, without added tuna	190	30	640
Tuna Salad (a)	1 cup	349	7.2	v
	1 lb	771	15.9	v
Tumeric, ground	1 tsp	8	1.43	1
Turkey, canned, meat only, boned	5½ oz can, solid pack	315	0	v
	1 cup	414	0	v
	1 lb	916	0	v
Turkey, cooked (roasted)				
total edible	8.6 oz, yield from 1 lb ready-to-cook	644	0	v
light meat without skin	1 cup not packed, chopped or diced	246	0	115
	1 cup not packed, ground	194	0	90
	1 lb (approx 3¼ cups chopped or diced, or 4⅛ cups ground)	798	0	372
	4 pieces (3 oz)	150	0	70
dark meat without skin	1 cup not packed, chopped or diced	284	0	139
	1 cup not packed, ground	223	0	109
	1 lb (approx 3¼ cups chopped or diced, or 4⅛ cups ground)	921	0	449
	4 pieces (3 oz)	173	0	84

Turkey Frozen Dinners
See Frozen Dinners, name brands
Turkey, potted
See Sausage, cold cuts, & luncheon meats

(a) Averages for salad prepared with tuna, celery, mayonnaise, pickle, onion & egg.

Food	Quantity or Portion	Calories	Carbo-hydrates (grams)	Sodium (milli-grams)
Turkey Giblets (some gizzard fat), simmered	1 cup chopped or diced	338	2.3	—
	1 lb	1,057	7.3	—
Turkey potpie, home baked	1 whole 9″ pie	1,654	129.1	1,906
	1 piece, ⅓ pie	550	42.9	633
	1 lb	1,075	83.9	1,238
Turnips				
raw, cubed or sliced	1 cup	39	8.6	64
cooked (boiled), drained	1 cup, cubed	36	7.6	53
	1 cup, mashed	53	11.3	78
	1 lb	104	22.2	154
Turnip Greens, leaves including stems				
raw	1 lb	127	22.7	—
cooked (boiled quickly), drained	1 cup	29	5.2	—
	1 lb	91	16.3	—
canned, greens & liquid	15 oz can	77	13.6	1,003
	1 cup	42	7.4	548
	1 lb	82	14.5	1,070
frozen, chopped, cooked (boiled), drained	1⅓ cups, yield from 10 oz frozen	51	8.6	37
	2⅛ cups, yield from 1 lb frozen	81	13.7	60
	1 cup	38	6.4	28
	1 lb (yield from 1.3 lbs frozen)	104	17.7	77

V

V-8 Juice
  See Beverages
Veal
  See also Frozen Dinners, brand names, for frozen Veal Dinners

Food	Quantity or Portion	Calories	Carbo-hydrates (grams)	Sodium (milli-grams)
Chuck cuts and boneless veal for stew, braised, pot-roasted, or stewed	8.4 oz, yield from 1 lb raw veal with bone	564	0	117
	10.6 oz, yield from 1 lb raw veal without bone	703	0	146
	1 cup, chopped or diced (not packed)	329	0	68
	1 lb	1,066	0	222
	1 piece (3 oz)	200	0	41
Loin cuts, braised or broiled	9.5 oz, yield from 1 lb raw loin with bone	629	0	174
	11.4, yield from 1 lb raw loin without bone	758	0	209
	1 cup, chopped or diced (not packed)	328	0	91

Food	Quantity or Portion	Calories	Carbo-hydrates (grams)	Sodium (milli-grams)
	1 lb	1,061	0	294
	1 piece (3 oz)	199	0	55
Breast of veal, braised or stewed	8.3 oz, yield from 1 lb raw veal with bone	718	0	108
	10.6 oz, yield from 1 lb raw veal without bone	906	0	137
	1 lb	1,374	0	207
	1 piece (3 oz)	258	0	39
Rib roast	8.5 oz, yield from 1 lb raw veal with bone	648	0	161
	11 oz, yield from 1 lb raw veal without bone	842	0	208
	1 cup, chopped or diced (not packed)	377	0	93
	1 cup, ground	296	0	73
	1 lb	1,220	0	302
	2 pieces (3 oz)	229	0	57
Round, with rump (roasts & leg cutlets), braised or broiled	8.7 oz, yield from 1 lb raw veal with bone	534	0	164
	11.3 oz, yield from 1 lb raw veal without bone	693	0	213
	1 cup, chopped or diced (not packed)	302	0	93
	1 lb	980	0	301
	1 piece (3 oz)	184	0	56
Vegetable Juice Cocktail, canned	6 fl oz can or glass	31	6.6	364
	24 fl oz can	124	26.2	1,454
	1 cup	41	8.7	484
	1 fl oz	5	1.1	61
Vegetables, Mixed (carrots, corn, peas, green beans, lima beans), frozen				
cooked (boiled), drained	1½ cups, yield from 10 oz frozen	176	36.9	146
	2.4 cups, yield from 1 lb frozen	285	59.6	236
	1 cup	116	24.4	96
	1 lb	290	60.8	240
Vegetable-oyster See Salsify				
Venison, lean meat only, raw	3 oz	107	0	—
Vienna Sausage See Sausage, cold cuts, & luncheon meats				
Vinegar				
cider	1 qt	134	56.6	10
	1 cup	34	14.2	2
	1 tbsp	2	.9	trace

Food	Quantity or Portion	Calories	Carbo-hydrates (grams)	Sodium (milli-grams)
distilled	1 qt	115	48.0	10
	1 cup	29	12.0	2
	1 tbsp	2	.8	trace

Vodka
  See Beverages

W

Waffles
  baked from home recipe, made with

enriched or unenriched flour	1 round waffle, 7″ diam, ⅝″ thick (yield from approx 7 tbsp batter)	209	28.1	356
	1 sq waffle, 9 × 9 × ⅝″ (yield from approx 1⅛ cups batter)	558	75.0	950
	¼ of above 4½ × 4½ × ⅝″	140	18.8	238
frozen, made with enriched flour, prebaked	12 oz container, 10 waffles, 4⅝ × 3¾ × ⅝″ each	860	142.8	2,190
	1 waffle	86	14.3	219
	5 oz container, 6 small waffles	359	59.6	914
	9 oz container, 12 small waffles	645	107.1	1,642
	1 small waffle (3½ × 2¾ × ⅝″ or 3¾ × 2¾ × ½″)	56	9.2	142

Waffle Mixes
  See Pancake & Waffle Mix
  See also Waffles, frozen, brand names

Waffles, made from pancake & waffle mix, with egg, milk	1 round waffle, 7″ diam, ⅝″ thick (yield from approx 7 tbsp batter)	206	27.2	515
	1 sq waffle, 9 × 9 × ⅝″ (yield from approx 1⅛ cups batter)	550	72.4	1,372
	¼ of above, 4½ × 4½ × ⅝″	138	18.1	343

Waffles, frozen, brand names
  Aunt Jemima Frozen Waffles

Blueberry	2 waffles	160	29	630
Buttermilk	2 waffles	170	29	700
Original Recipe	2 waffles	160	28	650

—133—

Food	Quantity or Portion	Calories	Carbo-hydrates (grams)	Sodium (milli-grams)
Downyflake Frozen Waffles				
Blueberry	2 waffles	180	32	570
Buttermilk	2 waffles	170	30	630
French Toast	2 slices	270	30	380
Original	2 waffles	170	30	500
Walnuts				
Black	1 lb in shell	627	14.8	3
shelled	1 cup	785	18.5	4
	1 tbsp	50	1.2	trace
	1 cup finely ground	502	11.8	2
	1 lb, yield from approx 4½ lb in shell	2,849	67.1	14
	1 oz	178	4.2	1
Persian or English	1 lb in shell	1,329	32.2	4
	10 lg nuts (approx 1⅝″ diam)	322	7.8	1
shelled	1 cup halves (approx 50)	651	15.8	2
	1 cup, chopped	781	19.0	2
	1 tbsp, chopped	52	1.3	trace
	1 lb (yield from approx 2¼ lb in shell)	2,953	71.7	9
	1 oz, approx 14 halves	185	4.5	1
Water Chestnuts, Chinese (matai, waternut), raw	1 lb	276	66.4	70
Watercress, leaves, including stems, raw	1 cup	7	1.1	18
	1 cup chopped fine	24	3.8	65
Water Ice				
See Ices, water				
Watermelon, raw	1 whole, 16″ long, 10″ diam, approx 33 lb	1,773	436.4	68
	1 piece, 10″ diam, 1″ thick, or ¼ piece, 4″ thick	111	27.3	4
	1 cup diced pieces	42	10.2	2
	1 lb cut pieces	118	29.0	5
Weakfish, broiled with butter or margarine	1 lb	943	0	2,540
	1 oz	59	0	159
Weight Watchers Frozen Dinners				
See Frozen Dinners, brand names				
Weight Watchers Frozen Desserts				
See Frozen Desserts				
Welsh Rarebit	1 cup	415	14.6	770
Wendy's				
Breakfast				
Bacon	2 strips	110	0	445
Danish	1 piece	360	44	340
French Toast	2 slices	400	45	850
Home Fries	103g	360	37	745
Breakfast Sandwich	129g	370	33	770

Food	Quantity or Portion	Calories	Carbo-hydrates (grams)	Sodium (milli-grams)
Eggs, Scrambled	91g	190	7	160
Omelets				
Ham & Cheese	114g	250	6	405
Ham, Cheese & Mushroom	118g	290	7	570
Ham, Cheese, Onion, Green Pepper	128g	280	7	485
Mushroom, Onion & Green Pepper	114g	210	7	200
Sausage	1 patty	200	0	410
Toast with Margarine	2 slices	250	35	410
Hot Stuffed Baked Potatoes				
Plain	8.8 oz (250g)	250	52	60
Bacon & Cheese	350g	570	57	1,180
Broccoli & Cheese	365g	500	54	430
Cheese	350g	590	55	450
Chicken a la King	358g	350	59	820
Chili & Cheese	400g	510	63	610
Stroganoff & Sour Cream	406g	490	60	910
Burgers				
¼ lb Single	118g	345(a)	23(a)	(b)
½ lb Double	197g	560	24	575
¼ lb Bacon Cheeseburger	147g	460	23	860
Chicken Sandwich	128g	320	31	500
Chili	8 oz	260	26	1,070
French Fries, salted, regular size	98g	280	35	95
Frosty Dairy Dessert	12 fl oz	400	59	220
West Indian Cherry **See Acerola**				
Wheat Flour, whole (from hard wheat)	1 cup stirred, spooned into cup	400	85.2	4
Wheat Flour, patent (white), plain				
All-purpose or family flour, enriched or unenriched	1 cup unsifted, spooned into cup	455	95.1	3
	1 cup sifted, spooned into cup	419	87.5	2
Bread flour, standard granulation, enriched or unenriched	1 cup sifted, dipped with cup	500	102.3	3
	1 cup sifted, spooned into cup	420	85.9	2
Cake or pastry flour	1 cup unsifted, dipped with cup	430	93.7	2
	1 cup unsifted, spooned into cup	397	86.5	2
	1 cup sifted, spooned into cup	349	76.2	2
Gluten flour	1 cup unsifted, dipped with cup	529	66.1	3

(a) Values differ slightly between multi-grain wheat bun and white bun.

(b) 290g sodium for multi-grain bun; 410g sodium for white bun.

Food	Quantity or Portion	Calories	Carbo-hydrates (grams)	Sodium (milli-grams)
	1 cup unsifted or sifted, spooned into cup	510	63.7	3
Self-rising flour, enriched	1 cup unsifted, spooned into cup	440	92.8	1,349
	1 cup sifted, spooned into cup	405	85.3	1,241
Wheat, parboiled				
See Bulgur				
Wheat Products used mainly as hot				
breakfast cereals				
Wheat, rolled	1 cup dry form	289	64.8	2
	1 cup cooked	180	40.6	708
Wheat, whole meal	1 cup dry form	423	90.4	3
	1 cup cooked	110	23.0	519
Wheat & malted barley cereal, toasted				
quick cooking (about 3 min cooking time)	1 cup dry form	517	106.0	1
	1 cup cooked	159	32.3	176
instant cooking (about 1 min cooking time)	1 cup dry form	439	87.6	1
	1 cup cooked	196	39.4	250
See also Farina				
Wheat Products used mainly as				
ready-to-eat breakfast cereals				
Wheat Bran				
See Bran				
Wheat flakes, added sugar, salt, iron, vitamins	1 cup	106	24.2	310
Wheat germ, without salt & sugar, toasted	1 tbsp	23	3.0	trace
Wheat, puffed				
without salt or sugar; added iron, thiamine, niacin	1 cup	54	11.8	1
with sugar or sugar & honey, & salt; added iron & vitamins	1 cup	132	30.9	56
Wheat, shredded				
without sugar, salt or other added ingredients	1 oblong biscuit, 3¾ × 2¼ × 1" or 2½ × ¼"	89	20.0	1
	1 round biscuit, 3" diam × 1"	71	16.0	1
	1 cup spoon-size biscuits, 50 biscuits	177	40.0	2
	1 cup crumbled biscuits	124	28.0	1
	1 cup finely crushed biscuits (3 oblong or 4 round or 1½ cups spoon-size)	266	59.9	2
with malt, salt, sugar; iron & vitamins added	1 cup bite-size sq	201	44.9	383
	1 cup shreds	146	32.7	279

Food	Quantity or Portion	Calories	Carbo-hydrates (grams)	Sodium (milli-grams)
Wheat & malted barley	1 cup flakes, added sugar, salt, iron, vitamins	157	33.7	226
	1 cup granules, without sugar; added salt, iron, vitamins	430	92.8	814
Whey	1 cup fl	64	12.5	—
	1 lb dried	1,583	333.4	—
Whiskey				
See Beverages				
Whitefish, lake				
raw	1 lb whole fish	330	0	111
	1 lb flesh only	703	0	236
baked	1 oz cooked (baked), stuffed	61	1.6	55
smoked	1 lb smoked	703	0	236
	1 oz smoked	44	0	15
White Sauce	1 cup thin	303	18.0	878
	1 cup med	405	22.0	948
	1 cup thick	495	27.5	998
Wild Rice, raw	1 cup	565	120.5	11
Wine				
See Beverages				

Y

Food	Quantity or Portion	Calories	Carbo-hydrates (grams)	Sodium (milli-grams)
Yam, tuber, raw	1 lb	394	90.5	—
Yambean, tuber, raw	1 lb	225	52.2	—
Yeast				
Bakers				
compressed	6 oz pkg, 1¼ sq piece	15	2.0	3
	1 oz	24	3.1	5
dry	¼ oz pkg (scant tbsp)	20	2.7	4
	1 oz	80	11.0	15
Brewer's, debittered	1 tbsp	23	3.1	10
	1 oz	80	10.9	34
Torula	1 oz	79	10.5	4
Yogurt				
See also Yogurt, brand names				
made from partially skimmed	8 oz container	113	11.8	115
milk	1 cup	123	12.7	125
made from whole milk	8 oz container	140	11.1	106
	1 cup	152	12.0	115
Yogurt, brand names				
Dannon Flavored Yogurts (a)	1 cup	260	49	95
La Yogurt, all flavors (a)	6 oz	190	32	90
Light 'N Lively, all flavors (a)	6 oz	160	30	92
Yoplait, all flavors (a)	6 oz	240	40	92

(a) Content may vary slightly according to flavor.

Food	Quantity or Portion	Calories	Carbo-hydrates (grams)	Sodium (milli-grams)

Yogurt, Frozen
  See Frozen Desserts
Youngberries
  See Blackberries

Z

Zwieback	6 oz pkg	719	126.3	425
	1 piece, 3½ × 1½ × ½″	30	5.2	18
	1 lb, approx 65 pieces	1,919	337.0	1,134